Young People, Housing and Social Policy

Edited by Julie Rugg

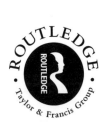

London and New York

First published 1999 by Routledge
11 New Fetter Lane, London EC4P 4EE

Simultaneously published in the USA and Canada
by Routledge
29 West 35th Street, New York, NY 10001

Routledge is an imprint of the Taylor & Francis Group

© 1999 Julie Rugg, selection and editorial matter;
individual chapters, the contributors

Typeset in Times by BC Typesetting, Bristol
Printed and bound in Great Britain by Clays Ltd

British Library Cataloguing in Publication Data
A catalogue record for this book is available from the British Library

Library of Congress Cataloging in Publication Data
Young people, housing, and social policy/edited by Julie Rugg.
      p.   cm.
Includes bibliographical references and index.
ISBN 0–415–18579–3. – ISBN 0–415–18580–7
  1. Youth–Housing–Great Britain.   2. Youth–Services for–Great
Britain.   3. Housing policy–Great Britain.   I. Rugg, Julie.
HD7333.A3Y68   1999
362.7'083'0941–dc21   98-50860
                                          CIP

ISBN 0–415–18579–3 (hbk)
ISBN 0–415–18580–7 (pbk)

Young People, Housing and Social Policy

While recent years have witnessed increasing interest in policy issues relating to young people, the issue of their housing needs has received scant attention. Presenting up-to-date empirical research on the subject of young people, housing and social policy in contemporary Britain, this book considers the issue of young people's early housing histories in the context of a range of government policy initiatives aimed at the group, and offers a critique of aspects of social policy that specifically address the housing of young people.

Young People, Housing and Social Policy provides new analyses of long-established datasets to give an up-to-the-minute account of young people and housing. Some chapters draw on data collected for specific housing studies, and others reflect on detailed interviews with young people themselves, so giving an intimate account of how young people experience a range of housing scenarios. It will be invaluable reading for students of social policy, welfare and youth studies as well as for policy makers with an interest in young people, housing and welfare.

Julie Rugg is a Research Fellow at the Centre for Housing Policy, University of York.

For my sister, Suzanne Blowey, for what she said
about editing books

Contents

Tables

Contributors

Isobel Anderson is a Lecturer at the Housing Policy and Practice Unit at the University of Stirling. She was previously a research fellow in the Centre for Housing Policy at the University of York.

Nina Biehal is a Senior Research Fellow in the Social Work Research and Development Unit at the University of York.

Roger Burrows is the Assistant Director of the Centre for Housing Policy at the University of York.

Bob Coles is a Senior Lecturer in Social Policy at the Department of Social Policy and Social Work at the University of York.

Janet Ford is the Director of the Centre for Housing Policy at the University of York.

Anwen Jones is a Research Fellow at the Centre for Housing Policy at the University of York.

Nicholas Pleace is a Research Fellow at the Centre for Housing Policy at the University of York.

Deborah Quilgars is a Research Fellow at the Centre for Housing Policy at the University of York.

David Rhodes is a Research Fellow at the Centre for Housing Policy at the University of York.

Julie Rugg is a Research Fellow at the Centre for Housing Policy at the University of York.

Jenny Seavers is a Research Fellow at the Centre for Housing Policy at the University of York.

Suzanne Speak is a Research Associate at the Department of Town and Country Planning at the University of Newcastle upon Tyne.

Jim Wade is a Senior Research Fellow in the Social Work Research and Development Unit at the University of York.

Preface

Victor Adebowale, Centrepoint

When reading this book I am reminded of Charles Dickens' opening line in *A Tale of Two Cities*: 'It was the best of times, it was the worst of times'. The chapters in this book describe in some detail the gaps, the prejudice and the adult world's sheer ignorance of what it is like to be young in today's society. It is largely this ignorance that leads to the sight of young people on the streets – not just in our major cities but also in towns and rural areas. In some ways, now is the worst time to be young. The pressure to be something, to make choices about your life, find housing and to become a citizen has never been greater. The pressure to succeed in an increasingly competitive society leaves those with what we call a 'disadvantage' way behind. Nearly a third of young people approaching Centrepoint for help have been 'looked after' in the care system. These young people continue to show up disproportionately in all the other misery statistics pertaining to crime, mental health, teenage pregnancy and of course drug misuse. The difficult transition from dependent childhood into independent adulthood is being made by too many young people without guidance, and without the essential bridge between the two that most people take for granted.

The fundamental safety net that should catch young people who end up on the streets is full of holes, and this books explains some of the ways in which our housing system fails young people. The welfare system is also failing to meet need, based as it is on the assumption that young people require less than the rest of us in order to survive. I am faced almost daily with stories of how young people arrive at our emergency shelters with no means of support. Even access to Severe Hardship Payments and Housing Benefit is restricted through demands for proof of identity (passports, household bills) and the suspicion that these young people are somehow attempting to rip off the state.

Young people who do access benefits are subject to the single room reference rent restriction on their Housing Benefit, which has resulted in private sector landlords simply refusing to provide accommodation to under-25s. We have a benefit system that assumes that the cost of living for a person under 25 is somehow less than that for someone over 25. The result is that young people who get work are faced with a steep drop in their Housing Benefit, which in many cases leaves them no better off after housing costs are taken from their wages. These benefit inequalities undermine the strong message to young people to get work through the New Deal. Such contradictions in government policies are only too obvious to young people, and contribute to the wider problem of their disillusionment with the democratic political process.

My introduction started with a quote from Dickens and an incomplete picture of the worst of times; but it is also the best of times. Why – because New Labour has used the language of youth in describing its vision for the future of Britain. In her first speech as Housing Minister, Hilary Armstrong used the occasion to state her commitment to youth housing and in particular to ending youth homelessness. The establishment of the Youth Homelessness Action Partnership (YHAP), in order to co-ordinate the activities of the youth homelessness sector, has given impetus to her commitment. The work of the Social Exclusion Unit in its first report on rough sleeping, and the interest of Gordon Brown in the fortunes of young people on New Deal, is a sure sign of a commitment to meeting the needs of vulnerable young people. The access given to the highest levels of government to youth homelessness agencies such as Centrepoint is further testimony to this commitment. In this respect we are living in the best of times. There has never been a better opportunity to persuade, cajole and influence those in power to make good their commitments. New Labour is asking for solutions, and I think there are some.

Understanding the needs of young people is essential in planning for real solutions in the prevention of homelessness. For example, as this book sets out, the causes of youth homelessness are complex but they are also no mystery. The causal factors of youth homelessness are known; young people are more likely to become homeless if they are poor; from an ethnic minority group; unemployed; suffer from a mental illness; come from a deprived neighbourhood or any one of the poorest local authorities; come from a family where the main breadwinner is unemployed; if they have been in care. Knowing these causal factors means that we can plot their prevalence in certain areas. Knowing the hot spots enables us to look at preventing youth homelessness by putting together often complex plans involving the voluntary, private, and statutory sectors in working together to provide integrated solutions to what is an interlinked problem. In other words, what works is a plan – not just any plan, but one that has been built in consultation with young people and which is based on a definition of the problem that they understand and agree with.

At Centrepoint we have been developing such plans for some time through our National Development Unit (NDU). In London we have an ambitious strategy to provide a city-wide prevention plan which has funding attached to its conclusions and recommendations. This Safe in the City plan is the first of its kind and I am hopeful that it will show the way in providing integrated solutions to the problem of youth homelessness.

Planning is one of the best ways of eradicating ignorance about the conditions under which too many young people live and sheds light on the reasons why they leave home chaotically. But a plan is not a safe place to stay in a crisis and is not enough money to live on. The need for a basic and fair benefits system must be a campaigning issue for those of us who are serious about meeting the housing needs of young people. Only this sort of state support can enable young people to compete in housing markets increasingly unresponsive to the needs of under-25s.

Acknowledgements

Many thanks are due to Jane Allen, Lynne Lonsdale and Margaret Johnson for their secretarial and administrative assistance in all the CHP-based research reported in this volume.

Almost all the chapters rest on research that could only be completed with the full co-operation of a range of statutory and voluntary sector agencies, and to these the authors express their gratitude. Principal thanks must, however, be given to the many thousands of young people who, in a range of different research contexts, have patiently answered questions in often exhaustive detail about their early housing careers.

Chapter 1

Setting the context

Young people, housing and social policy

Julie Rugg and Roger Burrows

This book aims to examine *housing issues* relating to *young people* within the broad context of contemporary debates within British *social policy*. This is a timely point at which to draw these three fields together, since the Labour government elected in May 1997 is in the process of defining its stance on a range of social and welfare issues; housing policy is in a state of flux as a consequence of a range of economic, political and cultural forces; and young people are increasingly being defined as a group requiring specific policy interventions. However, it is rarely the case that these three areas are considered in unison: for example, social and welfare changes are instituted for young people with only minimal recognition of the need to understand how these will interact with their ability to secure housing. The 'New Deal' for young people is perhaps a prime example, with employment policy makers only belatedly realising that young people need a secure housing base from which to hold down employment or training, and that restricted Housing Benefit payments to under-25s might undermine regulations encouraging young people to work. Similarly, broad housing issues are discussed without understanding that housing is an arena in which young people are particularly vulnerable: they often lack knowledge of their housing options; are frequently in low-paid and erratic work; and may not yet have the skills needed to negotiate positive housing outcomes for themselves. Thus, for example, policies that prioritise the allocation of social housing to families and older single people fail to acknowledge that young people are one of the groups least capable of competing for alternative housing in the private rented sector.

Where social policy debates have engaged with issues relating to young people and housing, the questions have tended to be bounded by a small number of relatively restrictive parameters. For example, books on young people sometimes include material on housing, but this material almost invariably focuses on a discussion of youth homelessness. The argument given generally reflects that young people are increasingly being viewed as an excluded group, with street sleeping being perhaps the most extreme manifestation of trends towards marginalisation in employment and benefits (for example, MacDonald 1998). Use of the concept of *transition* is also a common approach to dealing with young people and housing, and offers a valuable model to guide research. Within this literature, the transition from the parental home to independent living is usually analysed in relation to school to work transitions, and transitions from being a child to becoming a partner and/or a parent (A.E. Green *et al.* 1997). Gill Jones has completed extensive analyses of the concept of transitions and the early housing careers of young people leaving the parental home for the first time. This work has had an important impact in generating an understanding of the non-linear nature of this first move, with its false starts and subsequently necessary returns to the parental home (Jones 1995b).

The chapters in this volume pick up themes of marginalisation and underline the fact that youth homelessness remains a growing and pervasive problem which is likely to be exacerbated by structural forces within various housing markets. They also contribute to debates on youth transitions, and in particular discuss two instances – care leavers and lone parents – where transitions to independent living have been contracted and intensified, with a concomitant increase in the risk of failure and degree of vulnerability. The chapters also demonstrate the broad variety of housing circumstances experienced by young people early in their housing careers. However, in addition, this volume intends to provoke questions relating to the uses young people make of housing; and to examine in more detail areas that are sometimes hidden by the desire to construct overarching theoretical structures to contain young people's experience.

THE FAMILY, HOUSEHOLD AND HOUSING CIRCUMSTANCES OF YOUNG PEOPLE

This introduction begins the process of exploration by examining data produced through secondary analysis of the *Survey of English*

Housing 1996/7 (SEH). The data provide a statistical framework for introductory discussion, but also constitute a ready context in which to address broader issues and questions which later chapters will begin to address. The SEH is based on annual interviews with around 50,000 individuals living in around 20,000 households. Since April 1993 when the survey work began, a number of annual reports have been produced which discuss the SEH data collection; it is unnecessary to repeat that detail here (see Green and Hansbro 1995; H. Green *et al.* 1996, 1997, 1998). The SEH data for 1996/7 estimate that there were some 6,033,000 young people aged 16–25 living in households resident in non-institutional addresses in England. The following discussion does not therefore include statistics relating to, for example, students in halls of residence, or young people in prisons or hostels.

In order to understand the range of housing scenarios in which young people find themselves, it is perhaps useful to consider the nature of the groupings in which young people live. In housing terms, a distinction is usually made between a *family* and a *household*. In official surveys such as the SEH a family may be defined in one of three ways: it may be a married or cohabiting couple with no children; a married or cohabiting couple with children who themselves have never married; or a single person. A household may contain one or more families, and is generally defined as an address which is their main or only residence, and in which they have at least one meal together each day and share a living room. These definitions can usually cover most types of experience, but there are instances when housing situations become difficult to assess. For example, the sharing of accommodation is very common amongst young people and comprises a variety of experiences including lodging with another adult; living in a house in multiple occupation and sharing facilities with people who might not know each other, all of whom have separate tenancy agreements; and living in a house with a group of friends under some sort of joint tenancy agreement. In all these apparently different cases, the young person is judged as being a single-person family living in a single household.

Students represent another slightly problematic group. Under SEH definitions, students who live at home for only part of the year are not included in the data. Students living in halls of residence are also omitted because they have institutional addresses, and as a consequence the SEH data does not reflect this group. Students or any other young people regularly working part of their year away from the parental home are ambiguous in housing terms, and it may be that a new category needs to be created to recognise their particular characteristics. Ongoing work on young people in rural North Yorkshire found that students studying away from home themselves varied in their response to the question of whether they were living independently: some considered that being in the parental home during the long summer vacation meant that they had never really left. The study defined a category of 'student stayers' to take this type of experience into account (Coles *et al.*, this volume).

To facilitate discussion of young people in the SEH data, six mutually exclusive family circumstances have been defined:

- living in the parental home with two parents
- living in the parental home with one parent
- part of a couple with no children
- part of a couple with dependent child(ren)
- living alone without children
- living alone with dependent child(ren)

Table 1.1 gives a breakdown of the number and proportions of young people living in each of these circumstances. The data have been split by gender. The next few sections of the introduction will draw out the particular characteristics in young people fitting these categories.

Living in the parental home

The SEH 1996/7 found that living in the parental home is by far the most common housing location of young people, and was the situation of 3,552,000 (59 per cent) of 16–25 year olds. A common theme running through this book is the increasing pressure of structural forces encouraging young people to remain living in the parental home for longer (Coles *et al.*, this volume). A number of chapters point to economic, policy and housing market changes that have created difficulties for young people seeking to make their first steps towards independent housing. There is a close relationship between issues relating to living in the parental home and the substantial literature that has been produced on young people leaving home for the first time (Ainley 1991; Furlong and Cooney 1990;

Table 1.1 Family circumstances of young people aged between 16 and 25 in England, 1996/7

Family circumstances of young person	Males (000s)	%	Females (000s)	%	All (000s)	%
Lives in parental home						
With 2 parents	1,664	54	1,177	40	2,841	47
With 1 parent	420	14	291	10	711	12
Lives in a couple						
No children	284	9	477	16	761	13
With children	157	5	295	10	452	8
Lone adult						
On own	552	18	490	17	1,043	17
With children	9	0	217	7	225	4
Total	3,086	100	2,947	100	6,033	100

Note: Figures and percentages in this and subsequent tables in this chapter may not sum exactly due to the effects of weighting, grossing and rounding in the data. The source of the data in this and in subsequent tables is the SEH 1996/7, own analysis.

Jones 1990; Killeen 1992; Madge and Brown 1991). This material helps to explain the patterns of young people remaining at home. For example, the incidence of leaving home differs by age and gender: women are more likely to leave, and leave when they are younger, for the purposes of family formation (Jones 1990). As a consequence, it is more usual for men to be living at home with their parents than women: the SEH data showed only 50 per cent of female 16–25 year olds lived in the parental home compared with 68 per cent of men.

Reasons for leaving home are also associated with age: those leaving at aged 16–17 are likely to leave because of tension within the family; 18-year-olds most often leave to take up higher education courses; and later leavers are generally moving out to set up home with a partner (Jones 1990). Thus there are substantial age differences in the sub-group of young people remaining at home, and there is a marked decline in the proportion of home stayers as young people become older. According to the SEH, in 1996/7 almost 99 per cent of 16-year-old males lived in the parental home. By the age of 21 this percentage had reduced to 67 per cent, and at the age of 25 had dropped further to only 34 per cent. The

Table 1.2 Family circumstances of young men and women aged 16 to 25 in England in relation to the age of the young person, 1996/7

		Age of young person										
	Columns	16	17	18	19	20	21	22	23	24	25	All
Males												
Lives with parents	With 2 parents (%)	75	78	71	67	54	52	48	41	34	26	54
	With 1 parent (%)	24	19	21	16	13	15	8	7	7	8	14
Lives in a couple	No children (%)	0	0	1	2	4	8	14	16	19	22	9
	With children (%)	0	0	0	1	3	3	5	9	12	15	5
Lone adult	On own (%)	1	3	6	12	26	22	25	26	28	29	18
	With children (%)	0	0	0	0	0	0	0	0	1	0	0
Totals ('000s)		355	306	289	233	289	269	318	343	330	353	3,086
Females												
Lives with parents	With 2 parents (%)	76	73	61	46	36	35	33	19	17	12	40
	With 1 parent (%)	21	16	14	13	9	10	5	5	4	4	10
Lives in a couple	No children (%)	1	1	6	9	15	17	21	25	27	35	16
	With children (%)	1	0	2	4	5	7	13	16	23	25	10
Lone adult	On own (%)	2	7	12	20	27	26	21	23	17	13	17
	With children (%)	0	3	5	8	7	6	7	13	12	12	7
Totals ('000s)		303	293	282	246	267	291	282	341	305	338	2,947

reduction was even more marked in the case of young women: 97 per cent lived at home at the age of 16, dropping to 45 per cent at the age of 21 and only 16 per cent at the age of 25. Table 1.2 gives further detail. It becomes clear, therefore, that it is unwise to discuss 16–25 year olds as if they were a homogeneous group with a generalisable pattern of experience. Policy changes have been built on this assumption of homogeneity, and Rugg (this volume) discusses the introduction of a reduced assistance with housing costs for people under the age of 25 that was in part justified by the claim that most of this age group would still be living in the parental home.

Despite a detailed understanding of the reasons why young people leave home for the first time, and despite the fact that an extended stay in the parental home is increasingly well documented in statistical terms, the meanings of this shift in terms of family relationships have not yet been explored in depth. Even at a very basic level there will be differences in perceptions and expectations of a young person aged 16 and one aged 25 living in the parental home, as well as distinctions between young people who have never left, those who have left for a range of reasons and then returned for an equally broad set of reasons, and students who may spend up to three years living at home only for part of the year. Coles *et al.* (this volume) discusses the differences and the consequences for families meeting young adults' need for housing.

To add further complication to this question, it is evident that there are significant differences between groups of young people living in the parental home with two, and those living with one parent. The SEH data shown in Table 1.3 suggests that some 75 per cent of 16–25 year olds who live with their parents live with two parents. Some 82 per cent of young people in two-parent households lived in owner occupation whereas just 54 per cent of young people living with one parent did so. Almost 40 per cent of young people living with one parent lived in the social rented sector whereas just 14 per cent of young people living with two parents did so. To a large degree, the problematisation of young people living with lone parents – especially in social housing – has overshadowed the need for more qualitative research on related housing issues. Some research on the internal economic dynamics has been completed of families on low incomes where there is an adult child, and indeed some study has been made of the housing decisions of young people in families where their financial contribution could lead to a reduction in their parents' benefit entitlement

Table 1.3 Tenurial locations of young people in England aged 16 to 25, by differences in family circumstances, 1996/7

| Household tenure | Lives with parents | | | | Lives in a couple | | | | Lone adult | | | | All | |
| | With 2 parents | | With 1 parent | | No children | | With children | | On own | | With children | | | |
	(%)	(000s)	(%)	(000s)	(%)	(000s)	(%)	(000s)	(%)	(000s)	(%)	(000s)	(%)	(000s)
Owner occupation	82	2,333	54	386	57	431	42	191	27	286	10	23	61	3,650
Social housing	14	407	39	274	12	92	39	175	12	128	74	167	21	1,243
Private rented	4	101	7	51	31	238	19	86	60	628	16	35	19	1,139
Totals	100	2,841	100	711	100	761	100	452	100	1,043	100	225	100	6,033

(Kemp *et al.* 1994; Wallace 1987). In broader terms, it may be the case that there are differences in achieving independence from a single-parent family. Such a family may be less likely to be able to offer the financial support that young people often need to set up on their own, and perhaps less able to sustain a family home that young people could return to if they experience failure in their early housing career (Coles *et al.*, this volume).

Living as a couple

The SEH found that a total of 1,213,000 young people – 21 per cent – lived as part of a couple (Table 1.1). The gender differentiation is quite marked with respect to young people living with a partner. For example at the age of 16, the SEH recorded 2 per cent of women but insignificantly small numbers of men living as part of a couple. By the age of 21, 24 per cent of women and 11 per cent of men were living with a partner; at the age of 25 the differentiation had become more acute: 60 per cent of women were living with a partner, compared with just 37 per cent of men (Table 1.2). None of the chapters in this book directly address issues related to the joint early housing careers of young couples, but other studies have been completed. For example, Madge and Brown (1991) focused on young couples' movement around different tenures in the housing market. The SEH data suggest that young couples' early housing careers were shaped to a large degree by whether or not they had dependent children. The proportion of couples with children was small, although, as might be expected, this percentage did increase gradually with age. Compared with their childless peers, these couples were more than twice as likely to be living in social housing: only 92,000 (12 per cent) childless couples lived in social housing compared with 175,000 (39 per cent) couples with a child or children. It should be noted, however that 42 per cent of young couples with children – the majority of this group – were living in owner occupation, although in some cases this was because their household was 'nested' within another – usually headed by a relative of one of the young people.

Thirteen per cent of 16–25 year olds – 761,000 young people – lived as part of a childless couple. Most of these couples (57 per cent) lived in the owner occupied sector although some of these were living within other households – often where the head was not a relative of one of the young people. Few studies have addressed the housing needs of childless young couples, who may be considered to have advantages over single people within the housing market. For example, a couple is more able to rely on a dual income to finance entry into owner occupation. If the couple is on a low income, or reliant wholly on state benefits, sustaining a private sector tenancy may be easier. People who are living with a partner are not subject to restrictive Housing Benefit payments based solely on their age, and are likely to have all their private rental costs covered if they live in self-contained one-bedroomed accommodation that has a reasonable rent. In addition couples as a household type are generally favoured by landlords: even when couples have children, they are still preferred over single under-25 year olds (Crook and Kemp 1996). There are some indications that social housing is difficult for childless couples to secure: indeed, the SEH found as many lone young people as childless couples were in social housing (12 per cent). However, in general terms the SEH appeared to confirm that the great majority of young couples were able to secure independent housing. Over 95 per cent of couples – with or without dependants – lived in accommodation where the head of the family unit was also the head of the household.

Single-person households

According to the SEH, a total of 1,268,000 young people lived as lone adults outside the parental home and without a partner. As with couples and young people still in the parental home, there was some gender differentiation with respect to lone adults: there was a slightly higher proportion of young women compared with young men (24 per cent compared with 18 per cent), but the differentiation largely reflected the relatively high incidence of lone motherhood (7 per cent of lone women) compared with lone fatherhood (much less than 1 per cent). The different experiences in terms of gender also reflected in slightly different age distributions for men and women living as lone adults. Generally, the proportion of men living as lone adults increased gradually as they reached the age of 25: at 16, only 1 per cent of men lived alone; at 21 this proportion was 22 per cent; and at 25 the proportion had reached 29 per cent. Women, in contrast, reached a peak of lone adulthood at the early twenties then experienced a subsequent decline: at the age of 16, 2 per cent of women lived alone; at 21 this figure has reached

32 per cent, but by the age of 25 the proportion has dropped to 25 per cent (Table 1.2).

Again, as with young people living as couples, the housing experience of young lone adults depended to some degree on whether or not the young adult is a parent with a dependent child. The SEH found that 74 per cent of young lone parents – 167,000 young people, almost all of whom were mothers – lived in social housing. This sub-group of young people has been studied in detail (Burghes and Brown 1995; Clark and Coleman 1991). Single teenaged mothers were subject to intensive scrutiny in the latter years of the Conservative government, which for political reasons tended to exploit the myth of young women becoming pregnant to jump the social housing queue. However, recent research in this area has outlined the difficulties faced by young mothers in their attempts to establish a viable home, given lack of experience, limited support and often poor access to affordable good quality housing (Speak, this volume).

The vast proportion of young lone adults without dependants lived in the private rented sector. The SEH found that this was the tenure of 628,000 young people – 60 per cent – living alone. There is no gender differentiation amongst this group: on average 18 per cent of young men and 17 per cent of young women lived as lone adults. However, analysis of age differences again showed that men and women experienced different patterns of living alone without dependants. In particular, there was a marked decline in women without dependants living alone between the early and mid-twenties: at the age of 21, 26 per cent of young women are in this group, but by the age of 25 this proportion had halved to 13 per cent. To some degree, the declining number of young women living as single people in their mid-early twenties explains the gender bias in the increased incidence of housing need amongst young men – as evinced in a number of reports on single homelessness (Pleace and Quilgars, this volume).

Amongst the 1,043,000 young people who lived singly, only 320,000 (31 per cent) lived alone in a physical sense. The great majority – 723,000 – lived in either multi-person households or with relatives who were not their parents. Sharing accommodation is a common feature of young people's housing experience, and one that is only recently becoming the subject of exploration. The introduction of the Housing Benefit single room rent – with its implicit refusal to cover the costs of self-contained accommodation – has focused attention on the appropriateness of shared accommodation for young people (Griffiths 1997; Kirk 1997). Kemp and Rugg have questioned blanket assumptions about the vulnerability of young people in shared housing situations, and instead drew distinctions between different types of sharing. Many young people felt secure and happy to be sharing accommodation with a small group of friends or acquaintances, but were much less positive about living in larger houses with people who remained strangers and where everyone tended to sit in their room and not socialise (Kemp and Rugg 1998). According to the SEH, 84,000 young people who live with others live with relatives who are not their parents – for example, grandparents, aunts, uncles and other siblings. The range of experiences within this type of arrangement will vary considerably, from strong degrees of *in loco parentis*-type control to an experience close to that of sharing friends. The interaction between ties of obligation and any possible financial transaction becomes much more difficult to predict when young people are living with non-parent relatives. This type of kinship sharing has never been studied in detail from a housing perspective and may become more important as increasing reliance by young people on the parental home might begin to 'overspill' into a growing incidence of lodging with other relatives.

The housing of young single people outside of shared situations has become a burgeoning housing debate, particularly with respect to young single people on low incomes. Research in this area has tended to underline the fact that this group is remarkably homogeneous and requires housing providers and policy makers to meet a range of needs (Anderson and Quilgars 1995; Pleace 1995; Quilgars and Pleace, this volume). Indeed, this volume reflects the broad range of that debate in addressing the needs of young people leaving care, the Housing Benefit entitlement of single young people living in the private rented sector, and the particular problems faced by young people in rural areas in their attempt to secure housing. It is tempting to view young single people's housing entirely in terms of heightened or marginalised need, but there are degrees of ambiguity. For example, Rhodes (this volume) indicates that although cuts have been made in student financial support, they still maintain a position of strength in the private rented sector and often fare well in competition with other young people for rental accommodation.

Thus the sixfold household typology of young people living in the parental home (with one or two parents), living with a partner (with or without a child) and living alone (again, with or without a child) is a useful tool with which to explore the different housing situations of young people. The SEH data makes clear the fact that generalised presumptions about the housing needs and expectations of young people are untenable, and at the very least, gender and specific age have to be taken into account in framing policies for this age group.

ABOUT THIS BOOK

The chapters in this book are split into two sections. Section one includes three chapters which look at the three main housing tenures. Since owner occupation is the tenure of the great majority of the population, the volume begins with Ford's analysis of young people's experiences of entering into and sustaining home ownership. The chapter demonstrates that young people have begun to withdraw from this tenure. Indeed, it is possible to ask whether 16–25 year olds share the generally positive views held about owner occupation that have dominated British culture. It may be, rather, that young people are beginning to see mortgage payments and house maintenance as unsustainable burdens disproportionate to any advantages thought to attach to owner occupation.

Next, Anderson addresses the degree to which young single people can secure access to social housing. Where households are unwilling or unable to enter into owner occupation, renting from the council or from a housing association provides the most common alternative option. Anderson assesses local authorities' response to housing demand amongst young single homeless people, and indicates that access to housing can vary since local authorities have some discretion on the implementation of regulations. Even aside from basic differences between English and Scottish legislation on such issues as the age at which young people can hold tenancies, local authorities can choose the extent to which they can either prioritise or marginalise requirements to meet demand for housing from young people.

Both owner occupation and social housing might be considered 'lifetime' tenures: most people will spend the majority of their time in either tenure, and most of their moves will take place within their particular sector. Private renting – the third sector – tends to have a broader range of uses, as the chapter by Rugg demonstrates. This chapter discusses the use of the sector by young people both as a transitional tenure (prior to entry into home ownership or social housing) and a 'safety net', when entry to other tenures becomes difficult. Developments in assistance with private rental costs have failed to appreciate these uses of the sector, however, and have tended to problematise young people's reliance on private renting. Increasingly stringent restrictions have reduced assistance, on the assumption that young people would otherwise be induced to leave the parental home earlier than they would normally do so, or would live in high-rent accommodation at the taxpayers' expense. The chapter questions these assumptions.

The second section of the book takes as its focus the range of housing needs and experiences of 16–25 year olds. Rhodes's chapter looks in detail at the situation of students – an increasingly large sub-grouping – within the broader context of the operation of local housing markets. Rhodes recognises that the provision of housing for students has rarely been addressed. Their heavy reliance on the private rented sector means that their experience is subject to local differentiation, although for the most part students appear to be able to compete successfully for property in the sector.

By contrast, care leavers comprise a particularly vulnerable group. Biehal and Wade explain the way in which this group experiences very compressed transitions to independent living, often without the safety net of a possible return to the parental home. The chapter highlights the sometimes poor response of housing and social service departments to the needs of this group, and discusses elements of good practice in offering support and housing.

Young people leaving care often comprise a significant sector of the population of young homeless people. The chapter by Pleace and Quilgars addresses factors contributing to homelessness amongst young people, and uses large-scale datasets to define their characteristics. A following companion chapter (Quilgars and Pleace) looks in more detail at services designed to deal with youth homelessness and housing need.

Based on detailed qualitative work with a sample of young people in the North East, Speak discusses issues relating to the transition to independent living of lone parents. The chapter addresses the needs of both young mothers taking direct care of dependent children and young fathers who hope to continue having a relationship with their children despite being separated from the mother. The chapter indicates that transitional housing situations commonly used by young people are not appropriate to lone parents, who need access to stable, long-term housing close to sources of support.

Jones also looks at a group whose housing needs might be considered problematic: young people living in the countryside. The chapter demonstrates that features of the rural housing markets often disadvantage young people, who are subject to an exacerbated version of the difficulties with access to housing faced by their urban counterparts. Jones expresses caution about applying blanket assumptions relating to young people's housing requirements, and instead looks to the need for further research about young people's preferences and expectations.

The volume concludes with a chapter on young people living in the parental home. The chapter reflects Jones's caution with respect to generalisations about young people in a given housing scenario, and demonstrates that young people living with their parents comprise a group with a range of housing experiences and aspirations. The chapter looks at young people who have always stayed in the parental home, and those who have left and then later returned. Some attention is also given to young people who have yet to make housing decisions, and students' reliance on the parental home. The chapter draws out some housing consequences of an increased reliance on the parental home to house young people, considering its impact on the parents and family, and on the young people themselves. The conclusions are to some degree speculative, but do raise important issues that various of the contributors will examine in future research.

It must be recognised that these chapters by no means encompass the experiences of *all* young people's early housing careers. Nevertheless it is hoped that many of the broader questions raised by the chapters in this volume may help to frame housing research agendas for groups of young people not given explicit attention in this volume.

ACKNOWLEDGEMENT

Thanks are due to the Office of National Statistics (ONS) and the Department of Environment, Transport and the Regions (DETR) for agreeing to make available to us the SEH 1996/7 data files used in this chapter for secondary analysis. Much of the work in this volume was drawn together as background material to ESRC award no. L134251013 held by Janet Ford, Roger Burrows and Julie Rugg. The project, 'Young People, Housing and the Transition to Adult Life: Understanding the Dynamics' will report in 2001.

Chapter 2

Young adults and owner occupation

A changing goal?

Janet Ford

In recent times young people have played an important role in relation to owner occupation, which now encompasses 67 per cent of
households in Britain. In particular, they have been one key element
in its expansion to the current position as young people are an
important source of new households and so, potentially, of first-
time buyers in the housing market. The 1980s boom in 'starter
homes' was a physical and design manifestation of this relationship.
In turn, the increasing predominance of home ownership and the
associated reduction in opportunities to rent has led to a higher proportion of newly forming, young households moving into the tenure
as their first 'independent' housing destination and a reduction in
the time taken for all young home owners to reach that position
(A. E. Green *et al.* 1997). For much of the 1980s the evidence indicated that some of the strongest support for home ownership was
amongst young people up to the age of 35 (Kempson and Ford
1995), influenced by beliefs that it signified independence and
responsibility, conferred status and had the potential to generate
wealth. For young people, like others, owner occupation was
recorded as a desired and obtainable goal that increasingly signified
the completion of the transition to adulthood.

During the 1980s, the significance of home ownership for both
individuals and society was increasingly recognised as a focus of
analysis. For example, Saunders (1990) argued that home ownership
not only provided ontological security but also offered access to
wealth, and so the capacity to modify structures of inequality
through both widening access and the process of inheritance. On
this basis, the desire for home ownership amongst individuals in
general and young people in particular could be, and was, assumed.
Other perspectives, however, placed greater emphasis on the extent

to which the expansion of owner occupation was 'constructed', driven by ideological factors and fiscal incentives (Kemeny 1981; Forrest *et al.* 1990). Such accounts were also rather more critical of the likely outcomes of the expansion of home ownership. In particular, the uniformity of positive experience and assumed gains from owner occupation were challenged with evidence of and discussions about marginalised owners (Forrest *et al.* 1990) and failed ownership (Doling *et al.* 1989; Ford 1993). While these discussions were often about the inappropriateness of the tenure for households in particular circumstances, and so the need to provided either greater support for low income home owners and/or easier access to good quality rental accommodation, there was nevertheless an implicit acceptance of the assumption that, for whatever reason, and other things being equal, individuals' and households' preferences were to buy and own.

However, there are now both theoretical and empirical reasons to suggest that the relationship of people to home ownership may be changing and becoming more complex and less certain, and that some of these changes may be most pronounced amongst young people. At a theoretical level, writers concerned with the nature of societal change and its consequences in different ways, and for different reasons, point to the freeing-up, if not breakdown, of traditional structures and processes that until now have set the boundaries of activity and achievement and influenced the routes by which different groups of people move through the life course (for example, Giddens 1991; Beck 1992; Lash and Urry 1987). Thus, for example, Beck talks of the 'de-traditionalisation' and 'de-standardisation' of society, along with the suggestion that this offers individuals the opportunity (and responsibility) for greater self-determination and so the potential for a wider range of goals and diversity of pathways. Although infrequently discussed with respect to housing, this emerging perspective rather changes the questions and focus of research. Put simplistically, in relation to owner occupation, the central issue turns from the recent concerns with accepting the goal of owner occupation, and seeking to identify the barriers to its attainment (as discussed above), to one of seeking to identify whether or not, why, and under what circumstances owning a home becomes the desired housing goal. Issues of choice predominate, and while constraints are recognised they are not necessarily conceived as having social-structural roots.

But it is not necessary to accept the last theoretical perspective outlined above to recognise that empirically there is evidence that the traditional goals of young people with respect to housing may be changing. (There may also be changes amongst other groups, but this chapter is confined to young people.) Increasingly, young people face a series of wider social and economic changes that have the capacity to restructure the nature and speed of their transition to independent housing as well as to alter their preferred tenure (see, for example, Furlong and Cartmel 1997; Coles 1995). Some aspects of these changes may reinforce the existing relationship with home ownership (for example, increasing rates of both cohabitation and relationship dissolution, the reduction in social housing and an increasingly competitive private rented sector), while others may distance young people from owner occupation in the short and/or longer term (for example, the increasing proportion of young people in higher education, changes to student financing, the growth in labour market insecurity – particularly for entry jobs – and tighter credit referencing). While it is not inevitable, to a very considerable extent this stronger empirical focus has a preoccupation with constraints that emanate both from within the housing market itself and from the wider social, economic and political context.

This chapter explores three issues central to understanding the relationship between young people and home ownership. First, to what extent does owner occupation remain the desired goal of young people in the short and/or long term? Second, what are the key factors and structural changes shaping young people's decisions with respect to housing choice, and particularly owner occupation? Third, what has been the recent experience of young owner occupiers in terms of their ability to sustain their housing and at what cost? The discussion of these questions is, however, of an exploratory nature given the absence of detailed research directly focused on some of the pertinent issues, in particular detailed studies of the motivations underlying young people's housing decisions in the late 1990s.[1] A discussion of these issues is prefaced by a brief descriptive section on the current and recent pattern of young people in owner occupation.

The chapter considers the issues identified by drawing together findings from existing research. The principal definition of 'young people' used in this chapter is those between the ages of 16 and 24 (unless otherwise indicated), although it has to be recognised that this is an arbitrary cut-off point and many of the conclusions presented are likely to apply, at least to a degree, to those slightly older. This is increasingly the case as a range of social and economic changes act to extend the period of transition to adulthood (see for example, Coles (1995) for a general discussion, and Jones (1995b) and Ford *et al.* (1997) for a discussion of the extended nature of housing transitions). In any case, the 'transitionary end-point' has always been variable by socio-economic status (both that of parents and the young person) and gender, and, while less frequently considered, is also likely to be the case with respect to other variables such as ethnicity and disability.

YOUNG OWNER OCCUPIERS

According to Survey of English Housing 1996/7 data, the majority of the 5.3 million young people between the ages of 16 and 24 live in owner occupation (Rugg and Burrows, this volume). However, most of these are there by virtue of living with their parents who are owners. By contrast, in 1996/7 there were just 230,000 owner occupier households headed by a young person aged 16–24, although these households account for a larger number of young individuals. These owner occupier households comprised a quarter of all young independent households. Most were in the process of buying their homes with a mortgage. Table 2.1 shows the tenure distribution of young households and the household composition.

As a proportion of *all* owner occupiers, young households currently form only 2.5 per cent. However, 93 per cent of young owner occupiers in 1996/7 were first time buyers (6.5 per cent were repeat buyers and just 0.5 per cent – about a thousand households – purchased through Right-to-Buy), underlining their significance to the maintenance of the size of the market (H. Green *et al.* 1998). As a proportion of all first-time buyers in 1996/7, households headed by someone aged 16–24 formed around a quarter.

The figures in Table 2.1 are a snapshot of young independent households at a particular time. Time-series data show that the proportion of young people entering owner occupation, the proportion of owner occupiers who are young, and the proportion of young households in the first-time buyer population have all varied historically. For example, both the recent and current figures for the

Table 2.1 Tenure distribution of households headed by someone aged 16–24, by household composition, 1995/6 and 1996/97

Tenure	Marital status	Head of household, 16–24 yrs (000s)	All (000s)
Owned outright	Married	2	2,966
	Cohabiting	0	70
	Single	14	396
	Widowed	0	1,413
	Divorced or separated	0	279
	Total	16	5,124
Buying with a mortgage	Married	57	5,644
	Cohabiting	73	812
	Single	80	940
	Widowed	0	185
	Divorced or separated	4	852
	Total	214	8,433
Rented from Council	Married	25	1,134
	Cohabiting	38	225
	Single	108	654
	Widowed	0	838
	Divorced or separated	8	638
	Total	179	3,489
Rented from Housing Association	Married	8	286
	Cohabiting	11	52
	Single	46	217
	Widowed	0	208
	Divorced or separated	6	197
	Total	71	960
All private renters	Married	28	595
	Cohabiting	68	255
	Single	272	707
	Widowed	0	178
	Divorced or separated	6	294
	Total	374	2,029

Source: Survey of English Housing data 1995/6 and 1996/7

proportion of young households entering owner occupation are considerably lower than was the case in the 1980s. In part this is a reflection of the economic cycle, which is one influence on entry (and might help explain the lower entry figures in the earlier part of the 1990s, but less so in 1996/7), and in part a consequence of demographic factors (Holmans 1995a). However, there may also be shifts in attitudes and preferences shaped by wider structural changes and experiences that have impacted on young people in ways that have either limited their choices or led them to reassess their options. The next section considers the trend data in more detail in order to assess whether, and the extent to which, young people's commitment to owner occupation may be changing.

ENTRY TO OWNER OCCUPATION: CHANGING PATTERNS AND CHANGING ATTITUDES

Changing patterns

An important analysis by Alan Holmans (1995a), focused on the first-time buyer population, provides important insights into the issues of interest here – not least because, as already shown, young buyers are overwhelmingly first-time buyers. He shows for the age group of interest to this chapter that:

1   The proportion of any age group (16, 17, 18, etc.) making a first time purchase rose from 1974, fell in the early 1980s, rose again from 1983 and, while there was some variation by age, turned down substantially in 1989. Since then rates have fallen further, only starting to recover (marginally) in 1993. Data available since Holmans completed his initial analysis shows that this remained the position in 1996/7.
2   Whereas purchases have fallen in all age groups, the fall has been much steeper amongst young people. In those years where the overall number of first-time purchases showed some recovery, this was not realised to the same extent amongst younger age groups. This situation also persists.
3   Some of the fall in the proportion and number of young purchasers is due to demographic change in terms of the fall in the absolute number of people in each of the relevant ages. Some

of the downturn may also have been due to young people bringing forward purchases in the boom years of the mid-1980s, and
some to temporary delays associated with the housing market
recession of the early 1990s. However, notwithstanding these factors, there remains a continuing shortfall of young, new entrants
against the predicted levels, the reasons for which need to be
explored.

Changing attitudes

One potential explanation of the reduction in the proportion of
young people seeking owner occupation is that some reassessment
of the advantages and disadvantages of owner occupation has
taken place, resulting in a more cautious outlook. This may come
about in a number of different ways; for example, by the impact
of a change in the characteristics of ownership or by the impact of
a change in the circumstances of young people. Rising costs of purchase (stamp duty, estate agents' fees, etc.) might be an example of
the former, as might rising interest rates. Increasing youth unemployment or student debt, or a longer period of temporary,
poorly paid jobs in the early years of employment, might be
examples of the latter. Any change in the assessment of home
ownership may then be reflected in overall attitudes to home ownership or house purchase.

All the evidence shows that until recently there have been increasingly positive attitudes towards home ownership. Since 1976, the
Building Societies Association/Council of Mortgage Lenders have
commissioned a number of market research surveys designed to
measure changes in attitudes to home ownership. In particular,
respondents were asked to identify the tenure in which they would
most like to be living in two years' time (except in 1995 when the
question was not asked) and the one they hoped to be living in in
ten years' time. The ten-year preference question shows a historically
growing proportion of respondents wishing to be owners. Since 1986
the proportion has typically exceeded 80 per cent, although there has
been a downturn since the peak figure of 85 per cent in 1993 to 79 per
cent in 1996. Those aged 16–25 show the same broad profile as for all
respondents, but typically at a higher percentage figure. In 1989 the
overall figure was 83 per cent, but the figure for young people was
95 per cent. In 1996 the overall figure had dropped to 79 per cent,
while amongst young people it had dropped to 84 per cent – but

Table 2.2 Tenure preferences by age, 1983–97

| | Percentage of adults expressing a preference for living in owner occupation in 2 years' time | | | | | | |
	1983	1986	1989	1991	1993	1996	1997*
16–24	79	73	79	60	71	55	60
25–34	89	88	89	83	84	79	80
35–54	84	86	90	89	89	86	72
55–64	71	73	76	87	80	76	74
65+	56	61	64	71	72	66	60
All	77	77	81	77	81	77	73

Sources: British Market Research Bureau (1983, 1986, 1989, 1991, 1993), MORI (1996, 1997)

* Asked of those likely to move within two years

this was a lower figure than for those aged 25–34 and 45–54, indicating greater reservation/uncertainty amongst the youngest households. However, these findings have to be used cautiously given the very hypothetical nature of the question. Shorter-term attitude measures may therefore be a better indicator of likely behaviour, and Table 2.2 presents attitudes to owner occupation (measured by tenure preference in two years' time), disaggregated by age.

Table 2.2 shows the more volatile pattern of response amongst young people compared to other age groups. In addition, in the mid- and late 1990s young people have a much lower preference for home ownership than did 16–24 year olds in the mid- and late 1980s, notwithstanding the fact that unemployment has fallen since 1993 and the number of employment opportunities have increased. The table suggests that while support for owner occupation may be recovering as the economic cycle peaks, it has failed to return to the level associated with the peak in the previous economic cycle. These findings on attitudes are entirely in line with the findings reported earlier on patterns of entry to owner occupation.

Similar conclusions can be drawn from a number of other attitude surveys. The British Social Attitudes Survey, for example, has routinely measured attitudes to owner occupation by asking respondents to indicate whether they would advise a young couple with steady jobs to buy as soon as possible. Overall, fewer respondents advised them to buy as soon as possible in 1996 and 1997 than in 1986 (Murie 1997), and young people are the least likely to support this position (Ford and Burrows 1998). Further logistic regression analysis to examine the impact of a range of variables on attitudes to owner occupation (measured as outlined above) shows that age remains significant after controlling for the effect of other variables (Ford and Burrows 1998). Those aged 16–25 are less likely to recommend immediate purchase, even for those with steady jobs, than other age groups.

INFLUENCES ON ATTITUDES TO HOME OWNERSHIP AND HOUSING DECISIONS

Given the mounting evidence that attitudes to home ownership may be less positive than a decade ago, and that young people are now particularly cautious, at least over a two-year period, it is important to consider what factors are shaping these assessments. It has already been suggested that these influences are likely to emanate from the housing market itself, as well as from wider social and economic processes that are changing the circumstances of young people. There is not space to review the literature and statistics on the full range of changes that young people have experienced during the late 1980s and early 1990s. Rather, this section briefly identifies some important contenders and indicates the broad direction of change; it then goes on to discuss the evidence for their impact on young people's consideration of owner occupation.

In the decade from 1986 the housing market has been described as a 'roller-coaster', 'boom and bust' market. First-time buyers certainly experienced escalating house prices, rising interest rates and increases to their monthly mortgage payments at various points between 1987 and 1991. For example, annual increases in house prices in 1986, 1987 and 1989 were 15.6 per cent, 9.7 per cent and 19 per cent, respectively, based on sales to first-time buyers. Interest rates were around 11 per cent in 1987 and 1988 but rose to 13.6 per cent in 1989 and 15 per cent in 1990. Average monthly payments as a percentage of income for first-time buyers rose from £191 in 1986 to £398 in 1990 (Wilcox 1997). Some households also bought with 'low-start' financial deals which often lasted two or three years before they faced increases to their payments. If the end of the low-start period coincided with high interest rates, the increases were often very substantial indeed. Those who wished to exit the sector after 1989 found that prices overall were falling (although variable by region) and that potential buyers were limited as the number of residential transactions in England and Wales fell from 1.4 million in 1989 to just over 1 million in 1992.

With respect to young people, key texts consistently highlight the changing nature of provision and opportunities in the labour market (Ashton 1989; Roberts 1995), in education, and with respect to the provision of social security benefits (Rugg 1997), along with changing structures and preferences with respect to household formation and living arrangements (Jones 1990), changing patterns of dependency, leisure, consumption and lifestyle (Morrow and Richards 1996; Furlong and Cartmel 1997).

Many of these developments (for example, the restructuring of the labour market in a context of global competition and a policy response focused on deregulation) have resulted in increased youth unemployment, a greater likelihood of part-time, temporary employment and low wage employment. While the evidence indicates the life-time benefits accruing to those with higher education qualifications, even here a proportion (at times and in some subject areas quite a high proportion) of entry jobs are low skill and temporary (Steel and Sausman 1997). The expansion of higher education and the shift from grant to loan funding for students are also significant changes, with implications for the transition to adulthood in the form of financial independence and independent housing.

Other key changes relate to patterns of household formation, both the timing and their nature. There is evidence of greater cohabitation amongst young people, but also a considerable level of relationship failure. Young people also experience change as a result of parental household dissolution and re-formation as single parent households or step-parent households which can then be a spur to young people to find independent housing.

Potentially, a wide range of changes are likely to have contributed to the findings of a number of surveys that have shown consistently over the 1990s that a higher proportion of people have perceived owner occupation as 'risky', and that this is particularly pronounced amongst younger households. Risk is associated both with the costs of home ownership and with the perceived insecurity of the labour market (BMRB 1995; Murie 1997; Ford and Burrows 1998). These perceptions have particular implications for young people and are likely, at the least, to lead them to consider carefully the timing of any entry to owner occupation. What is more difficult to know currently is whether and how far the perception of owner

Table 2.3 Reasons for not entering the housing market

| | 18–24 | 25–35 | All unlikely to buy in the next two years |
	(n = 128) (%)	(n = 100) (%)	(n = 475) (%)
Employment situation	23	41	26
Properties too expensive	16	17	12
Need to save/cannot save for deposit	37	33	25
Unable/unwilling to take on mortgage debt	24	38	31
Would find it difficult to keep up with mortgage payments	14	27	18
Costs of buying are too high	19	17	13
Renting is flexible	11	18	11
Too young	44	6	13

Source: BMRB (1995)

occupation as a valued goal has altered such that even in the absence of structural constraints and insecurities owner occupation would be eschewed.

Table 2.3 presents the results from a survey in 1995 that asked all current non-owners (i.e. potential first-time buyers) reporting that they were *unlikely* to enter the housing market in the next two years why this was so. The major response categories for 18–24 year olds are presented and, for interest, the comparable percentage figures for those aged 25–34 and for all respondents. Table 2.3 confirms that both housing market conditions and wider social and economic change are important in shaping housing decisions. In particular, the costs of owning and current labour market circumstances are influencing young people's decisions. Almost a fifth of those aged 16–24 were unlikely to buy because of the costs of buying. Roughly one in seven thought property was too expensive, while a similar proportion thought they might have difficulties paying the mortgage. Not unconnected to this, almost two-fifths indicated that they had not yet saved, or could not save, enough for a deposit. Approaching a quarter indicated that their employment position precluded entry. A quarter were unwilling or unable to take on debt, an issue that potentially links to the growing number of higher education students and their exposure to debt (see Rhodes, this volume) but might also reflect the low wages available to many young people in entry jobs and the above average levels of unemployment amongst 16–24 year olds. By far the largest percentage, however, noted that they would be unlikely to buy because they were 'too young', suggesting that one interpretation of their current position might favour the view that their caution is less about owning *per se*, but more about owning under the right circumstances.

Some evidence in support of this possibility comes from a recent study of the housing destinations of a cohort of graduate students (Rosser 1997). Graduates provide an interesting lens through which to look at young people's changing attitudes and decisions about owner occupation because traditionally they have had access to good jobs, careers, and compared to many other groups of young people this is still the case (Roberts 1995). They therefore provide a test of changing attitudes and behaviour amongst one of the most favourably placed groups of potential entrants to owner occupation. They are also a significant group because they are growing in number and currently form around 40 per cent of the first-time buyer population. Any reluctance to purchase on their part might be indicative of even greater reluctance amongst other first-time buyers. They are also interesting because their position may be changing, as since 1990 they have been leaving higher education with a growing level of debt as first the maintenance grant was frozen and subsequently abolished and student loans were introduced. Some commentators, for example Maclennan *et al.* (1997) argue that as these changes progress even further they are likely to depress entry to home ownership significantly, although there are other views that are perhaps more equivocal (Laslett 1998).

In his study, Rosser (1997) traced the housing destinations of a cohort of students who had graduated between 1991 and 1995, seeking particularly to assess the impact of increased student loans and fear of falling property prices (a key characteristic of the housing market in the early and mid-1990s). In the first year following graduation, owner occupation was confined to mature students who were owners prior to entering higher education. Most graduates returned to the parental home even though they were typically employed. Only three years after graduating (aged 24 or over) did the rate of owner occupation increase, and five years after graduation 75 per cent were mortgagors. Ownership was closely tied to living with a partner. Amongst those who did not buy, potential labour market mobility (chosen or imposed) was a major factor, as was low income in relation to house prices, although this was less prominent. Student debt was not a significant deterrent to owner-ship in this study, although the author raises the possibility that in the post-Dearing regime it may become a larger issue. Using a different methodology, a not dissimilar conclusion is reached by Laslett (1998) – at least with respect to the short-term impact of student debt – and again the preferred interpretation of young people's likely behaviour is one of deferred entry rather than a rejection of the tenure.

YOUNG PEOPLE AND SUSTAINABLE HOME OWNERSHIP

Earlier sections of this chapter have shown how the proportion of young people entering home ownership shrank in the 1990s and discussed some of the reasons why this came about and is currently being sustained. One important influence was a growing belief that owning was 'riskier' than previously, but young people also believed that, for a range of reasons, it was less attainable. In contrast to the focus on the reluctance or inability to enter the tenure, this section explores the experience of those who did become owners. These two issues might also interconnect. To the extent that the experience of owning was problematic, and recognised more widely as such, potentially it could reinforce the perception of home ownership as a risk.

Most young owners in the early and mid-1990s will have entered home ownership in the late 1980s. Some may have been encouraged into home ownership by the buoyant, rising market, a fear that their ability to enter was diminishing monthly and the provision of double tax relief (MIRAS) which, it is claimed, led to a surge of young entrants in the three-month period before its pre-announced abolition in August 1988. In general, as already noted, rising house prices increased the amount borrowers needed to borrow. In turn, this increased their monthly repayments, while the deregulated and highly competitive mortgage market provided the necessary loans and, in addition, offered a number of discounted products to ease entry amongst those on the margins. The development of the housing market in the 1980s is well documented and need not be repeated here (see for example, Forrest *et al.* 1990; Forrest and

Murie 1994; Ford 1997). The cessation of double MIRAS was claimed to have encouraged unrelated young adults to get together ('to buy at speed and repent at leisure'), as well as encouraging those intending to buy as couples to enter sooner than they might otherwise have done.

By late 1989, for a range of reasons (for a full discussion see Forrest and Murie 1994), interest rates had started to rise and transaction to slow. In the early 1990s the downturn in the housing market became pronounced as prices continued to fall, giving rise at one point to over a million cases of negative equity whereby borrowers found that their property was worth less than the value of their outstanding loan; entrants in the late 1980s were most exposed to equity shortfall. An increasing number of borrowers either found it difficult to meet their monthly payments or were unable to do so, fuelled in large part by unemployment and reduced income from employment amongst mortgagors (Ford *et al.* 1995b). At the height of the housing market recession more than a million home owners were in arrears of at least two months; between 1990 and 1995 over 250,000 households lost their homes through the possession process, while one in five mortgagors experienced some payment difficulties between 1991 and 1993 (Ford *et al.* 1995b).

Young people were amongst those most at risk of arrears and possessions. Tables 2.4a and 2.4b present data from the Survey of English Housing on the percentage of households in arrears or experiencing payment difficulties, by age, for four years 1993/4–1996/7. Prior to 1993, age-specific data on arrears was only available from one-off studies. The best estimate for 1992 is that 6 per cent of those aged 16–24 had arrears of three of more months (Ford and Wilcox 1992).

Table 2.4a Percentage of mortgage arrears by age, 1993/4, 1994/5, 1995/6, 1996/7

Age of head of household	1993/4	1994/5	1995/6	1996/7
18–24	7	4	0	3
25–34	7	5	5	4
35–44	7	5	5	4
45–54	5	4	4	3
55–64	3	3	3	2
65+	3	2	4	1

Source: SEH data 1993/4–1996/7

Table 2.4b Percentage with payment difficulties by age, 1993/4, 1994/5, 1995/6, 1996/7

Age of head of household	1993/4	1994/5	1995/6	1996/7
18–24	14	11	11	14
25–34	12	13	13	11
35–44	17	14	13	13
45–54	14	14	13	11
55–64	15	11	11	13
65+	14	17	7	13

Source: SEH 1993/4–1996/7

For mortgagors aged 18–24, arrears peaked at 7 per cent in 1993 when one in every 13 young mortgagor households, missed payments. A further 14 per cent, or one in every six young borrower households, found it difficult to pay. Altogether, in 1993, more than one in five of young households found their mortgage problematic in some way. Only one age group had a higher level of problems: the 24 per cent amongst those aged 35–44. Amongst those aged 25–34 and 45–54 the figure was 19 per cent, with lower figures for the older age groups.

However, arrears fell more rapidly amongst young households in 1994/5 than was the case for other age groups (where in some cases default increased), and in 1995/6 no cases of arrears amongst the youngest age group were recorded by the SEH. It is possible that the percentage drop in arrears was, in part, a consequence of the higher rate of possession amongst young households and, in part, a consequence of the tighter credit screening by lenders that was instituted for all new borrowers from about 1991 onwards. The suggestion about the role of possessions, though, is quite difficult to investigate via the available national survey data. However, one earlier study of properties taken into possession by a large national lender in 1991 noted that 10 per cent were from those aged 21 and under, with a further 47 per cent taken from those between the ages of 22 and 29 (Ford 1993). Possessions were over-represented in both age groups compared to their share of all mortgagors. The same study also indicated that voluntary possession was particularly high amongst young households and included a small number of cases where borrowers had 'walked away' from the property even in the absence of arrears. The particular lender concerned perceived the higher levels of arrears and possessions, and particularly voluntary possessions, to be influenced by the lower level of commitment to home ownership amongst young people, particularly those who had bought with an unrelated other in order to obtain the advantage of double MIRAS (see p. 29). Voluntary possession was also likely to have been a result of not having to wait for a court order in order to secure local authority rehousing, given that households without children (many of which are young households) have no eligibility for rehousing. This drop in arrears was, however, relatively short-lived and by 1996/7 arrears amongst young people had reappeared when 3 per cent (approaching 6,500 households) had missed payments.

The extent of payment difficulties also fell amongst young people in the mid-1990s, but increased again in 1996/7 when almost 30,000 young households reported that while they were making their mortgage payments they were only doing so with difficulty. In 1996/7, young people reported a higher percentage level of difficulty than any other age group, although not the largest percentage increase in difficulties, these occurring amongst those aged 65 plus. Thus as concerns grow about the imminence of the next economic recession, young mortgagor households are already at considerable risk, and even more so than most other age groups.

It is of course quite possible that what appear to be differences in arrears and difficulties by age are merely manifestations of the impact of other variables. Analyses using logistic regression have been undertaken in order to examine the impact of a range of variables, including age, after controlling for all other variables. Age remains significant in increasing the odds of arrears and difficulties with younger borrowers more likely to develop arrears than older borrowers.

As already indicated, mortgagors have faced difficult conditions in the housing market in the late 1980s and 1990s. Despite this, when asked to indicate whether or not they were pleased that they had bought their present accommodation (which could have been recently or many years ago), the overwhelming majority were (86 per cent). The majority of these purchasers would have had many years of 'asset growth' to set against the 1990s downturn. However, amongst those aged under 30, one in seven regretted their purchase (H. Green et al. 1998). By definition these were all households who bought post-1985, many of whom would have entered on rising prices, faced rising interest rates and mortgage payments, and then the housing market collapse. While a wide range of factors potentially influence their assessment of home ownership, it is likely that housing market conditions themselves contribute to their disaffection with the tenure.

THE IRON CAGE OF HOUSING POLICY

There is clear evidence that fewer young people are entering owner occupation and that a substantial proportion are cautious about the tenure. Some recognise that if they wanted to buy at a young age they would find it difficult to do so and hard to sustain. Some have tried and failed. An answer to a key question – whether what we are recording is a temporary downturn structured by housing market constraints, a permanent shift to delayed entry structured by a wide range of constraints or a more permanent reassessment of tenure preferences, or, as is more likely, some combination of these processes – is not possible yet, although there is evidence in support of the first two of these three possibilities.

Any more permanent reassessment of tenure on the part of young people, however, raises the issue of its relationship to current housing policy. Successive governments since the late 1970s have made clear their commitment to owner occupation alongside their reluctance to support social housing other than for those in severe need. This overall pattern remains the policy direction of the Labour government elected in 1997, although there is a stronger commitment in principle to maintaining, improving and supporting social housing and social housing communities. With respect to home ownership, the language has changed from that of its further expansion to a concern with its sustainability, but no real reduction in the proportion of households in owner occupation is envisaged. Much is said about the need to support and expand the private rental sector, and there is general recognition that it remains a critical linchpin in the housing system, but policy initiatives are few and fiscal support and initiatives are deemed inadequate to bring about much additional investment (Kemp 1997).

From a policy perspective, the scope which young people have to 'choose' an alternative tenure on a permanent basis, if this is what they want to do, looks severely limited. Housing policy is a major constraint on the possibility of realising 'de-standardisation' and 'de-traditionalisation'. In the absence of alternatives, all that most young people can do currently is to delay their entry until the pressure for independent living leads them to 'accept it' in order to secure other valued objectives such as partnership, family formation, privacy or adulthood. Thus delayed entrants might include reluctant owner occupiers as well as those with a preference to own but whose entry has been constrained by the range of social, economic, institutional and educational changes already discussed. Currently the balance between these groups is unclear and research is necessary to explore the motivations and preferences for housing in order to identify the extent and direction of any change. A key task for policy makers is to develop a sensitivity to the changing preferences and to modify policy accordingly.

NOTE

1 An ongoing study is addressing this issue. 'Housing Transitions and Young People' is being undertaken by the author with colleagues from the Centre for Housing Policy at the University of York. This study will explore the form and reasons for the housing decisions and housing careers of young people in all tenures and address directly their perspectives on owner occupation.

Chapter 3

Young single people and access to social housing

Isobel Anderson

In order to complete the transition from youth to adulthood, albeit an extended or fractured transition, young people require access to a secure, affordable, long-term home. Since the late 1980s, young people aged 16–24 have been over-represented among single homeless people (Anderson *et al.* 1993) and much subsequent research and analysis on youth housing issues has focused on homelessness (Hutson and Liddiard 1994); special initiatives such as foyers (Quilgars and Anderson 1997; Anderson and Douglas 1998); private sector access schemes (Rugg 1996, 1997); and 'Rough Sleepers' initiatives (Randall and Brown 1993, 1995, 1996). Much less attention has been paid to young people's opportunities to secure more permanent housing in the social rented sector.

Recent research into single people's access to social housing (Anderson and Morgan 1997) found that young people faced significant barriers in finding more permanent solutions to their housing problems. The study sought to assess how single people of working age (without dependent children) faired in the social housing system and whether outcomes varied for different groups of single people, such as young people (aged 16–24). The research involved analysis of a sample of local authority and housing association policy documents; a postal survey of all local authorities in Scotland, England and Wales; and multi-agency case studies in five local authority areas. The data was collected prior to implementation of the 1996 Housing Act for England and Wales, the implications of which are discussed towards the end of the chapter. It had been hypothesised that local providers would have implemented positive policies to tackle the youth housing and homelessness problems of the 1990s, but the study confirmed that young single people remained among those most disadvantaged in the systems which determined access to social housing.

SOCIAL HOUSING: THE IMPORTANCE OF THE ACCESS PROCESS

The social housing sector comprises the housing stock owned and managed by local authorities (and some other public bodies), housing associations and, increasingly, other registered social landlords (Balchin 1995; Currie and Murie 1996; Williams 1997). Patterns of housing tenure vary across Britain and change over time. In 1995, local authorities accounted for 18.9 per cent of the housing stock in Britain, with housing associations making up 4.4 per cent of the total (Wilcox 1996). The main geographical variation was in Scotland where councils owned 31.1 per cent of the housing stock in 1995 (Wilcox 1996).

Debates on the nature of social housing have been increasingly interpreted in relation to residualisation of the stock and marginalisation of the tenants, relative to other tenures (Forrest and Murie 1983; Malpass and Murie 1994). More recently, these trends have been associated with the concept of social exclusion (Berghman 1995; Lee et al. 1995; Lee and Murie, 1997). While the term 'social exclusion' remains controversial and contested, there is a degree of consensus on two associated characteristics. Social exclusion is taken to be 'more than poverty' embracing a *comprehensive* analysis of disadvantage in the social, economic, political and cultural spheres (embracing exclusion from housing). Social exclusion is also taken to be *dynamic* rather than static, and there has been concern amongst researchers to identify the key *processes* which create or sustain social exclusion (Room 1995). A detailed critique of the debates on residualisation and social exclusion is beyond the scope of this chapter, but the notion of *process* aids the analysis of the housing element of young people's transition to adulthood. That is to say, in order achieve secure housing in the social sector, potential tenants must successfully negotiate the access process.

Social housing traditionally catered for the working classes, and increasingly housed those on the lowest incomes (Malpass and Murie 1994). The process of gaining access to social housing is determined by legislative and bureaucratic procedures, rather than by the free operation of the market. Within a national, statutory framework, local housing providers have considerable discretion as to who is eligible for housing. Throughout the 1980s and 1990s most providers aimed to allocate vacant properties according to the needs of those who applied for housing, and most did this by means of a housing waiting list and a set of procedures by which applicants were awarded priority on the list (Anderson and Morgan 1997). Local housing authorities also had statutory duties towards homeless households (Robson and Poustie 1996). Young single people who apply for social housing will, therefore, be in competition with older single people and other households for available properties. Young couples or young parents may be treated differently in the access procedures, especially the homelessness procedures, hence the specific consideration of single young people in this chapter.

A considerable body of research has previously been conducted into the process of access to housing (Venn 1985; Prescott-Clarke *et al.* 1988; Parker *et al.* 1992; Evans *et al.* 1994; Prescott-Clarke *et al.* 1994; Lidstone 1994; Withers and Randolph 1994; O'Callaghan *et al.* 1996; Mullins *et al.* 1996; Britain and Yanetta 1997). Many of these studies focused either on homelessness or on the waiting list and either on local authorities or housing associations, rather than undertaking a comprehensive review of all access routes into social housing. Only Venn (1985) focused specifically on the experiences of single people and none looked in detail at the position of young single people. While there were valid reasons for the specific research objectives and questions in these preceding studies, Anderson and Morgan (1997) sought to look at the policy and practice of local authorities and housing associations towards single people, across all access routes. The research method allowed policy and practice towards young single people to be identified and compared with that towards other household types.

HOUSING NEED AND DEMAND

If social housing providers are to allocate vacancies according to *need*, they have to define and measure the housing needs of households in their areas of operation. The matter of whose needs should be met by social housing has evolved over the years according to prevailing social trends and political ideologies. That is to say, access is dependent upon some measurement of housing need (inadequate housing circumstances) and a value-based judgement as to the legitimacy of an individual's or household's claim for assistance.

Successive government statements have emphasised state responsibility towards *families*, rather than to all citizens (Holmans 1995b). Consequently, questions have been raised as to the legitimacy of young people's expressed demand to form independent households, and to obtain secure housing in the social sector if they cannot afford to buy or rent in the private market. Furthermore, the housing needs of young single people have tended to be neglected in national estimates for social housing provision, such as those provided by Whitehead and Kleinman (1992) and Holmans (1995b). Young single people seem to be viewed as 'individuals who are not yet families' and thereby do not require the same security and independence in their housing as family households. Garside (1993) similarly argued that such attitudes resulted in the assumption that single people were adequately housed in temporary, shared accommodation.

Local housing authorities have a statutory responsibility to assess housing needs within their areas as part of their strategic and enabling role (Goodlad 1993, 1994; van Zijl 1993). Nearly three-quarters (73 per cent) of local authorities surveyed for Anderson and Morgan (1997) attempted to identify the housing needs of single people, including young single people. However, qualitative interviews confirmed that assessing need was problematic and that there may be substantial numbers of young single people whose housing needs were not accurately reflected in local assessments. This was sometimes because they did not register on the waiting list or apply for help if they were homeless, and sometimes because other methods for assessing housing needs did not fully take account of young single people.

Available local authority information indicated that single people in housing need comprised a diverse range of individuals with varying social characteristics and needs, who experienced a wide range of housing circumstances. Nevertheless, single people's housing needs were commonly characterised by a high degree of insecurity in their housing situation, sometimes to the point of moving around between different addresses or sleeping out. Patterns of insecurity and housing need often reflected factors such as lack of privacy, overcrowding and difficult relationships with families or landlords.

Some single people also had particular health-related needs and support needs. Although the growth in the number of single people aged under 25 years was expected to slow down, housing providers still viewed this age group as one which continued to place high demands on social housing (Anderson and Morgan 1997).

THE COUNCIL HOUSING LIST

Queuing on a 'waiting list' has been the traditional route into council housing, although, for England and Wales, the Housing Act 1996 replaced waiting lists with unitary housing registers. In managing the housing list and the allocations process, local authorities set criteria which governed registration on the list, eligibility for allocations, and priority on the list. A wide range of criteria were employed and some were of particular importance in relation to the housing opportunities for young single people.

Under Scottish legislation, all young people were eligible to apply for council housing and to hold a tenancy from the age of 16 years. In England and Wales, however, age restrictions on eligibility to join the housing list and to be allocated a tenancy often discriminated against young people. The critical differentiation was between the treatment of those aged 16 or 17 years and those aged 18 and over. Only half of English and Welsh authorities allowed 16-year-olds to register on the housing list, and nearly a third denied

Table 3.1 Age at which applicant may join the housing waiting list

| Age (years) | Household type | | |
	Single person (% of LAs)	Couple (no children) (% of LAs)	Household with children (% of LAs)
16	53	51	63
17	6	7	6
18	38	42	31
19+	3	0	0
Total	100	100	100
N	133	131	128

Source: Postal survey of local authorities (Anderson and Morgan 1997)

Table 3.2 Age at which applicant may be allocated a property

	Household type		
Age (years)	Single person	Couple (no children)	Household with children
	(% of LAs)	(% of LAs)	(% of LAs)
16	34	31	43
17	2	3	2
18	60	65	55
19+	5	1	0
Total	100	100	100
N	127	125	122

Source: Postal survey of local authorities (Anderson and Morgan 1997)

Note: Percentages may not sum exactly due to rounding

access to households with children where the parent was less than 18 years old (Table 3.1).

The restrictions placed upon young people were even more severe when it came to being allocated a property (Table 3.2). In some areas, while young people could join the waiting list at 16 or 17 years, they did not normally become eligible for a tenancy until they reached 18 years of age. Only one-third of authorities said single people and couples were eligible for rehousing at age 16, while just over two-fifths said this was the case for households with children. Where local authorities did allocate tenancies to applicants under 18 years of age, over three-fifths said they would require a guarantor for rent or other tenancy matters, reflecting their legal status as minors.

Once registered on the housing list, young single people were in competition with other applicants for available lettings. In determining the relative priority of different applicants, local authorities typically awarded points for a wide range of factors. The higher the number of points awarded to an application, the greater the likelihood of being offered a tenancy. The research found, however, that these needs-based points systems often neglected those factors most likely to apply to young single people. For example, only half of councils took account of the applicant being in hostel accommodation and less than half took account of non-statutory homelessness, rooflessness, or insecurity of accommodation.

LOCAL AUTHORITY HOMELESSNESS DUTIES

Since its introduction in 1977, the homelessness legislation has excluded most young single people from the priority groups who are entitled to housing. Young single people who applied for assistance under the homelessness provisions would only be entitled to housing if they were found to be homeless (and not intentionally so) and in priority need on account of vulnerability due to special reasons. While people aged 60 years and over are awarded priority on account of their age alone, this has never been the case for young people despite their much higher probability of experiencing homelessness.

Local authorities have a considerable degree of discretion in making decisions with regard to whether young homeless people are vulnerable and, consequently, in priority need of accommodation. For example, they could operate a discretionary policy of accepting young people in certain age groups as being vulnerable, but Anderson and Morgan (1997) found that few chose to do so (Table 3.3). Only a quarter of authorities always or usually accepted young people aged 16–17 years as having priority need, and only 10 per cent did so for 18–24 year olds, with little difference in practice towards 18–21 year olds compared to 22–24 year olds (Table 3.3).

Homeless young people's access to council housing may also be influenced by social services legislation. The Children Act 1989 and the Children (Scotland) Act 1995 placed duties upon social services and social work authorities with respect to young people who had been in care or were considered to be otherwise in need

Table 3.3 Whether age alone was accepted as affording homelessness priority need

Age (years)	Always/usually accepted (% of LAs)	Sometimes accepted (% of LAs)	Never accepted (% of LAs)	Don't know (% of LAs)	N
16–17	26	56	14	4	185
18–21	10	46	32	12	184
22–24	10	38	37	15	182

Source: Postal survey of local authorities (Anderson and Morgan 1997)

Table 3.4 Whether care-related circumstances were accepted as affording single homeless people priority need

Care circumstance	Always/usually accepted (% of LAs)	Sometimes accepted (% of LAs)	Never accepted (% of LAs)	Don't know (% of LAs)	N
Care leaver age 16–17	49	40	8	3	182
Previously in care (not immediate care leaver) age 16–17	22	65	9	4	185
Care leaver age 18	29	57	10	4	184
Previously in care (not immediate care leaver) age 18–21	7	71	15	7	184
Young person referred under the Children Act (England and Wales only)	51	36	7	6	154

Source: Postal survey of local authorities (Anderson and Morgan 1997)

(McCluskey 1993, 1994; Corbett 1998). The Children (Scotland) Act 1995 was implemented after the data collection period for Anderson and Morgan's (1997) study, but data was available for English and Welsh local authorities. Around half of authorities always or usually awarded priority to young homeless people who were care leavers aged 16–17, and to those referred by social workers under the Children Act provisions (Table 3.4). Young homeless people who had been in care but were 18 or older at the time of application, or who applied some time after leaving care, were treated much less favourably.

Two-thirds of local authorities in England and Wales who responded to the survey said they had a joint working agreement between housing and social services in respect of Children Act referrals (Anderson and Morgan 1997). Less than half of those authorities were able to give information on the number of young people they had permanently housed in the previous year under the terms of the Children Act – and the average number of allocations was only four tenancies in the year. Local authorities were even less receptive to awarding priority-need status in other circumstances which were relatively common among young homeless people. Few councils recognised the associated problems resulting from drug/alcohol abuse, having been in prison (or youth detention), or rooflessness as indicators of vulnerability under the homelessness provisions (Anderson and Morgan 1997).

HOUSING ASSOCIATIONS

Housing associations do not have the same statutory duties towards homeless households as local authority housing departments. However, they often use needs-based points systems to determine priority for housing and usually allocate half of all vacancies to applicants nominated by the local authority. Anderson and Morgan (1997) found that housing association policies were generally more sensitive to the needs of young single people than those of local authorities. For example, most allowed young people to apply for a tenancy, and to be allocated their own place, from the age of 16 years. Typically, housing association allocation policies took reasonable account of insecure housing situations, and they often prioritised those who were roofless and other homeless households who did not fall within the precise priority categories of the homelessness legislation. During most of the 1990s, however, central government exerted pressure on associations to house statutorily homeless households, rather than young single people.

Despite expansion during the 1980s and 1990s, associations accounted for less than 5 per cent of the housing stock in 1995 (Wilcox 1996) and the sector could not be expected to meet all of the demand from young single people. As the social rented sector continues to diversify through the transfer of council housing to other landlords (Mullins *et al.* 1992, 1995; Taylor with Wainwright 1996) it will become increasingly important to monitor the opportunities for young single people to gain access to housing provided by a large number of new agencies.

ALLOCATING AND MANAGING TENANCIES

Decision-making in the day-to-day allocation process was illustrated in the case study examples in Anderson and Morgan (1997). Young single people competed with other household types for all except the smallest vacancies. Allocation practice in one case study area (a metropolitan borough council) revealed how young single people faced informal, as well as formal, barriers in gaining access to a tenancy. Staff in local housing offices made decisions about who was allocated vacant properties, although the overall policy was set centrally. The largest and fastest growing demand for housing came from young single people. However, an evident factor which contributed to the relative disadvantage of single people was the practice, by some area offices, of designating *mature-person* blocks of flats. This meant that younger single people were denied access to otherwise suitable vacancies, through the entrenchment of local practice rather than central policy (Anderson and Morgan 1997: 59).

For those young people who successfully secured a social housing tenancy, problems sometimes arose in managing in their homes. While tenancy problems occurred among a range of household types, young single people were sometimes more likely to be perceived as 'problem tenants' by social landlords. Landlords reported that individual young people often experienced tenancy 'failures' due to rent arrears, 'anti-social' behaviour, or, simply, not being able to manage on their own. Where a high proportion of young tenants were concentrated in particular blocks of flats or areas of lower demand housing, then the sum of individual problems could have a wider impact on the local community.

The difficulties experienced by young single people in managing in independent tenancies reflected the *comprehensive* dimension of social exclusion, as experienced by many young people in housing need. Gaining access to secure housing did not overcome the disadvantage they experienced in the labour market and the social security system, which meant they had to get by on very low incomes. Similarly, a secure home did not necessarily resolve the problems some faced as a result of their childhood experiences, estrangement from their families, isolation or lack of independent living skills.

The perception that young single people may become 'problematic' tenants also influenced their chances of being offered accommodation in the first place. More than half of the local councils surveyed said that offers of accommodation to young single people were sometimes conditional upon the provision of support by some other agency (Anderson and Morgan 1997). For example, where applicants were leaving care or had been referred under the Children Act legislation, there might be a requirement for social work support in the new tenancy.

Despite the acknowledgement that young single people faced a range of potential difficulties in managing tenancies, only two-fifths of local authorities surveyed said that they provided support to young or vulnerable single people to assist them in their new homes. The support provided mainly involved housing managers liaising with other agencies on behalf of tenants, with few authorities employing specialist resettlement or support workers, or providing furnished tenancies. More recent research has indicated that where local authorities have provided furnished, or part-furnished accommodation, there have been benefits for both landlords and tenants (Harding and Keenan 1998).

THE HOUSING ACT 1996 AND SUBSEQUENT POLICY DEVELOPMENTS

The Housing Act 1996 (Part VII) repealed the homelessness provisions of the 1985 Housing Act for England and Wales and set out new procedures. The main change introduced was that where a household was deemed unintentionally homeless and in priority need, the authority's duty would be to secure accommodation for up to two years, rather than the more permanent duty accepted under the earlier legislation. Statutorily homeless households would be placed in temporary housing and required to wait for an allocation of social housing through the new unitary housing register, also introduced in the 1996 Act (Irvine 1996). The new Act was unlikely to enhance the opportunities for young single people to gain access to social housing as it did not incorporate any substantial changes to the groups considered to be in 'priority need' in the event of homelessness. Some further guidance was given on the special vulnerability of young people aged 16 or 17 years, but there was still no priority entitlement to housing for this age group.

The new Housing Act also amended the other criteria by which English and Welsh local authorities could allocate their housing.

In particular, section 161 of the 1996 Act required authorities to allocate housing only to people who were defined as 'qualifying persons', including persons over 18 years of age owed a duty under the homelessness provisions. The requirements within the Act that local authorities give consideration to people occupying temporary or insecure accommodation, or with a particular need for settled accommodation, were potentially helpful to young single people. However, authorities retained discretion in the structuring of their schemes (for example, in setting relative priorities through points systems for allocations), and the entrenched discrimination against young single people, especially those aged 16 or 17 years, was likely to continue.

The impact of the changes in practice had not, however, been evaluated at the time of writing. Preliminary findings from a study by Pawson and Third (1997) suggested that, in practice, many authorities were awarding substantial rehousing priority points to applicants threatened with the loss of accommodation or living in insecure accommodation. In some instances, this meant that homelessness in the sense of the previous legislative regime was actually avoided. Pawson and Third acknowledged that their early conclusions would require confirmation through a more rigorous, representative study (Pawson and Third 1997).

In May 1997, the new Labour government announced proposals for amendments to the implementation of the Housing Act 1996 (*Inside Housing*, 30.5.97). Although the legislation was not changed, the government stipulated that households accepted as statutorily homeless would be included as a category on the housing register, to which authorities should give preference in the allocation of secure housing. The government specified that suitable accommodation for homeless households should be available for a period of at least two years. These amendments were subject to a consultation period ending on 20 June 1997, with implementation from late 1997. The changes went some way towards restoring the position which pertained under the Housing Act 1985 for priority homeless households, but did not alter the disadvantageous position of young single people.

Following the implementation of the Housing Act 1996, the homelessness provisions for England and Wales differed from those in operation in Scotland for the first time since 1977. After the 1997 election, the Scottish Office produced a revised code of guidance on homelessness which strengthened the guidance on good practice in implementation of the homelessness legislation (Scottish Office Development Department 1997a). The new code of guidance emphasised prevention of homelessness (particularly rooflessness) through local strategies and provision of adequate emergency services. In assessing vulnerability of young homeless people, Scottish local authorities were encouraged to take expert advice and exercise sympathetic discretion (Scottish Office Development Department 1997a). In a separate amendment, a new category of priority need (due to vulnerability) was introduced from January 1998 (Scottish Office Development Department 1997b). Young people aged under 21 who had been in care or looked after by a local authority at age 16, were to be included within the priority need groups in the event of homelessness. This marked an important departure from the discretionary position which pertained in England and Wales.

During 1998, the Cabinet Office Social Exclusion Unit was set the task of developing a strategy to reduce street homelessness in England. The Unit's first report on rough sleeping made a number of recommendations on the treatment of young single people within the homelessness procedures (Social Exclusion Unit 1998). Although the tone of the proposals was potentially helpful for young single people, the detail left ultimate discretion with local housing authorities. For example, the report suggested that care leavers *with very few exceptions* should be accepted as vulnerable, and that homeless 16- and 17-year-olds who have no social support should *normally* be regarded as vulnerable (Social Exclusion Unit 1998). There was no further discussion as to why there should be exceptions in practice, or what circumstances might warrant such exceptions. Similarly, the report recommended that local authorities should develop effective strategies to prevent homelessness (Social Exclusion Unit 1998), but made no mention of ensuring fairness in access procedures.

POLICY OPTIONS FOR THE FUTURE

If young single people on low incomes are to achieve independent living as part of their transition to adulthood, access to secure, affordable accommodation must be a realistic prospect. Transitional accommodation such as foyers and other supported housing can play a valuable role in times of crisis and in preparing young people for independent housing. Eventually however, many young people will look to socially rented housing as a long-term option, increasingly so as access to the privately rented sector is curtailed through Housing Benefit restrictions. While it would be naïve to suggest that a council or housing association tenancy could be a simple solution to the complex problems experienced by many homeless and badly housed young people, a fairer chance at establishing a secure base would represent a fundamental starting point.

Anderson and Morgan (1997) suggested a number of practical measures which could be implemented quickly to ensure that young single people received more equal treatment in the procedures which determined access to social housing. Firstly, local authorities and housing associations in England and Wales could be legally required to allow all young people to register for council housing and to hold a tenancy from the age of 16 years. This policy could be implemented, along with a broader move towards a common age of majority for young people, at age 16, across social policy areas. The current situation where young people cease to be 'children' in terms of social services provision at 16 years, but do not become 'adults' in terms of housing legislation until they reach 18 years, is contradictory and highly unsatisfactory. Moreover, this anomaly has undoubtedly been a contributory factor to the high incidence of homelessness amongst young people, especially those leaving the care system. While that contradiction prevails it follows that all homeless young people aged 16 or 17 years, and all young people deemed 'in need' under the Children Act legislation, should be included in the statutory priority need groups under the homelessness provisions.

National government could also place a firm duty upon social housing providers to give specific consideration within their allocation priority schemes to the range of insecure housing situations experienced by young single people. In addition, when young single people are offered housing, this should be accommodation of a reasonable quality in an area where they will have, at least, a chance of making a success of their tenancy. Young single people, like other applicants for social housing, need to be given a reasonable degree of choice in the allocations process if sustainable communities are to emerge.

Beyond these initial measures, consideration could be given to increasing the priority, within the allocations process, to young single people who have drug and/or alcohol dependency problems;

are, or have been, roofless; were formerly in local authority care, but are no longer 'in the system'; or were formally in prison or youth detention. Experience of these situations can be very damaging to young people and they may well behave disruptively or require intensive support in order to get by in their own home. Such difficulties have been well documented, but the resources available for tenancy support have proved inadequate (Anderson and Morgan 1997).

Whether tenancy support is a legitimate landlord role or should be taken on board by community or social work agencies, or in multi-agency partnerships, is a matter for debate (see, for example, Deloitte and Touce Management Advisory Service (1997) for a discussion of the 'Housing Plus' concept in the housing association sector). What matters is that the need for earmarked funding for support services must be recognised. Central government and local service providers could make a substantial difference to the long-term housing outcomes for young people by prioritising support services for independent living and by finding the additional resources needed to fund those services.

Finally, tackling youth unemployment and youth poverty are fundamental to improving the quality of life of disadvantaged young people. If initiatives such as the New Deal for young un-employed people (Department for the Environment, Regions and Transport, Welsh Office and Scottish Office 1997) are to succeed, the importance of stable and secure housing must also be a priority in the welfare to work strategy. At a time when some local authorities, particularly in the north of England, are reporting excess supply in relation to demand (Holmes 1998), local authorities and housing associations could make an increasingly valuable contribution to meeting the housing and support needs of young single people. Providers need to adopt flexible policies which respond to long-term social trends. The dismantling of exclusionary barriers to the access process could enable young single people to play a more constructive role in social housing communities of the future.

NOTE

This chapter builds upon earlier work: Anderson (1997) and Anderson and Morgan (1997).

Chapter 4

The use and 'abuse' of private renting and help with rental costs

Julie Rugg

Britain is a nation of owner occupiers: taken as a whole, 68 per cent of the population live in property that is either owned outright or in the process of being paid for through a mortgage. In societal terms, owner occupation is a cultural norm, the history and meanings of which have been examined extensively (Saunders 1990; Dupuis and Thorns 1998). Young Britain, by contrast, is a nation of renters. Secondary analysis of the Survey of English Housing data shows that 60 per cent of single people aged 16–25 – 628,000 individuals – live in the private rented sector (PRS) (Rugg and Burrows, this volume). However, the use of private renting by young people is an area that has been infrequently addressed. For example, even at a very basic level there is uncertainty about the proportion of young people who may be termed 'willing renters' who have made a choice in favour of that tenure, and about how many young people have simply ended up renting for want of any viable alternative. The issue of choice and constraint is particularly marked for young people reliant on state benefits, a group that will be the focus of this chapter.

Many young people on benefits use private renting as either a transitional tenure or residual housing. These uses are reliant to some degree on the availability of state support with rental costs. However, since the mid-1980s a gradual shift in policy has taken place: it is now considered that only some types of renting arrangement are appropriate for young people, and Housing Benefit regulations have been altered accordingly. The chapter discusses the rationale for changes in policy, in which the desire to cut welfare spending is often underlined by questionable assumptions relating to young people's 'abuse' of their benefit entitlement, drawn on to duck parental control and move into over-expensive accommodation in the private rented sector. At the heart of this particular issue is the degree to which the availability of help with housing costs impacts on housing decisions, and the chapter outlines the difficulties relating to the assessment of claimants' behaviour. The chapter concludes with offering some comment on the way in which changes in policy have affected the ability of young people to use the PRS as either a transitional or residual tenure. The chapter begins by an explanation of these two uses of private renting.

FUNCTIONS OF THE PRIVATE RENTED SECTOR

In their analysis of private renting in the mid-1980s, Bovaird *et al.* (1985) identified four main functions of the sector, including the provision of short-term housing for the 'young and mobile'. Bovaird *et al.* made no distinction between the young and the mobile, but analysis of 1980s National Health Service registration data showed that youth and mobility were closely connected. The 16–24 year old age group moved far more often than other age group, with those in their twenties being particularly mobile (Rosenbaum and Bailey 1991). The private rented sector also served the purpose of housing those unable to secure accommodation in other sectors. This renting sub-group largely comprised single people on low incomes.

For the purposes of this chapter, it is these uses of the sector that have most importance: its purpose as a 'transitional' and 'residual' sector are both uses closely associated with young private renters. Transitional renting may be defined as an interim letting arrangement, with the housing used for short periods of time. This kind of private renting is often associated with life events such as leaving the parental home or separating from a partner. The renter intends to stay in the sector for perhaps a couple of years, during which time there may be a number of moves from one rented situation to another. For young people at early stages in their housing careers, this period in a transitional sector before finally entering a lifetime tenure of either social housing or owner occupation may be mirrored both by movement around the labour market and eventual settling into work, and the process of finding a partner and perhaps beginning a family.

Transitional use of the PRS is encouraged by a number of factors. First, relative to the other tenures, it may be possible to get in and out of private renting quickly. Buying a home necessitates a complex process of negotiating a mortgage, dealing with solicitors and arranging surveys; and entry into social housing sometimes requires the accumulation of priority points – often through a long wait on a housing register. Securing a place to rent can – if the tenant is lucky – take little more than a day, if a vacancy is available and the landlord is willing to let immediately. Second, letting arrangements are such that young people can enter into tenancy agreements for periods as short as six months, and after that time has elapsed can give as little as a month's notice to quit. By contrast, moving out of owner occupation is by no means a speedy affair, since it can take some time to secure a buyer before being able to move on to other accommodation. Third, the ability to secure furnished accommodation means that young people are not tied down with the expense and inconvenience of moving around furniture and white goods such as freezers and washing machines.

The sector also fulfils the function of a residual sector. Again, this use is particularly associated with the young, and especially young people on low incomes. Chapters in this book have described ways in which young, single people are excluded from the lifetime tenures of social housing and owner occupation (Ford, Anderson, this volume). It is unnecessary to reiterate here the degree of young people's exclusion from these tenures, aside from commenting that by the process of elimination the PRS then becomes the most viable housing option. The PRS also operates as residual housing in the sense that it is often viewed as providing accommodation in which people would not actively choose to live. The domination of an owner-occupation culture means that private renting in particular is viewed principally in terms of its disadvantages. For example, Marsh and Riseborough's recent discussion of private renting hinged on the way in which the citizenship rights of private renters tended to be eroded, despite the existence of tenancy and quality regulation (Marsh and Riseborough 1998).

Many of the features of the PRS which make it so amenable for use as a transitional tenure also mean that it can act, equally well, as a residual tenure. For people on low incomes, ease of access may also connote affordable access. Landlords – particularly of bedsits and houses in multiple occupation (HMOs) – are sometimes willing to let accommodation on payment of rent in advance alone,

with a limited deposit or a deposit paid in instalments. The availability of furnished accommodation in the PRS is also important
for young people early in their housing careers, whose incomes
may not be high enough to cover for savings for or loan repayments
on furniture and white goods. In addition, privately rented accommodation – like social housing – removes from the tenant the
responsibility for property repairs and maintenance.

Bovaird et al. (1985) indicated that both lifetime use of the PRS
and tied renting were in decline, but demand for rented accommodation as transitional and residual housing would be dependent on
economic trends and housing policy. This conclusion – drawn as it
was in the mid-1980s – was correct. Both economic developments
and consequent housing policy initiatives have had a substantial
impact on the use made by the sector of young people on low
income. The chapter will continue by demonstrating this case, focusing on changes that have been made to young people's entitlement to
assistance with private rental payments.

YOUNG PEOPLE AND ASSISTANCE WITH PRIVATE RENTS

Up until the 1980s, age was not taken into account when deciding
eligibility for help with private rental costs. The shift to a differential
system, begun in the mid-1980s, has taken place over three main
stages which have applied gradually tightening restrictions, reducing
the amount of assistance a young person may receive. This section
will outline three major benefit changes: the establishment of benefit
time limits for under-26-year-olds in board and lodgings; the
abolition of the householder/non-householder distinction; and the
introduction of the single room rent.

Board and lodgings payments

During the mid-1980s changes were made to housing assistance for
people living in board and lodgings. This help was delivered as the
Housing Benefit component of Supplementary Benefit, and its
maximum was assessed by the local benefit officer as being the
equivalent of 'a reasonable weekly charge'. From April 1985, the
ability to set a local maximum was removed, and board and lodgings
payments became subject to a national ceiling of £50–60. A slightly

higher level was set for Greater London. In addition, further regulation established a time limit on the period during which people under the age of 26 would be eligible for the payment. Again, there was a regional difference on the limit: young adults would be paid for either two, four or eight weeks depending on the area in which they lived. The shortest time period applied to young people living in certain coastal areas. After that time had elapsed, unless the young person had moved on to alternative accommodation, the Supplementary Benefit would no longer include the additional amount for board and lodgings (Matthews 1985; Harris 1989). It should be noted that these payments have now been abolished.

The abolition of the 'householder' distinction

Within months of the introduction of the time limit on board and lodgings payments for under-26s, a second and more radical change was announced. The Green Paper published in June 1985 proposed the abolition of the householder/non-householder distinction (Secretary of State for Social Services 1985a). It had been the case that differential housing assistance was given according to whether the recipient was a householder. It was assumed that certain people – for example, those living in the parental home – would have lower housing costs compared with people who had the responsibility for maintaining a home, and so would require a reduced level of assistance. The 1985 Green Paper introduced a new, age-based differential, and specified that lower payments would be made for young people under the age of 25. The regulation change took no account of young people living independently in the private rented sector, who would receive a lower rate of benefit than someone over the age of 25 living in the same type of accommodation. As with the board and lodgings payments, these regulations have since been abolished.

The Green Paper also signalled the introduction of Housing Benefit. This payment – made separately from any welfare supplement to income – was implemented from April 1988. Although it was not intended that Housing Benefit itself should – at this stage – be used to deliver a restricted assistance to under-25s, the interaction of the benefit's complex regulations with new limits placed on young people's levels of Income Support means that in some cases young people on low incomes receive restricted assistance compared with those over 25 (Kemp 1992). At the time of writing, this anomaly still operates.

The introduction of the single room rent

The third revision further refining housing assistance for young people was the introduction of the single room rent (SRR), enacted through the Housing Benefit (General) Amendment Regulations 1996 (S.I. 1996 No. 965). This change did carry the direct objective of reducing housing assistance for young renters, by limiting Housing Benefit payments to the level of the average rent for a 'single room' in that locality – the single room rent. All young single people without dependants in private rented accommodation – with some limited exceptions – would be paid at or below the same rate, no matter what their housing circumstances. For example, an under-25-year-old living in a single person flat and being asked for a rent of £65 would only be paid the equivalent rent of an average room in a shared house with access to shared bathroom and kitchen facilities (but no living room), which may only be £35. The recipient would be expected to meet the shortfall of £30 from their own resources, move, or negotiate a lower rent (Kemp and Rugg 1998). At the time of writing (1998), this regulation is still in force.

Thus, it can be seen that the history of assistance with private rental costs is essentially one of gradual restriction, to the degree that it is now the case that young single people in the PRS are only likely to have their rent fully covered by benefit if they live in very basic rooms in shared housing. The next section explores the rationale proposed for these changes, examining the way in which the desire to cut welfare spending has been underpinned by some-times overt misrepresentation of young people's housing behaviour.

THE RATIONALES FOR CHANGE

For many commentators, much of the explanation for increasing restrictions on the level of housing assistance given to young private renters rests with economic factors (for example, Harris 1989). Historically, it has always been the case that where economic trends push down employment rates, welfare budgets are contained by implementing cuts and ensuring a more exact targeting of resources. This trend was a feature of the boom/bust years of mass unemployment in the 1920s and 1930s, when increasingly stringent restrictions were placed on the eligibility for assistance of those people who were out of work (Thane 1989). The late 1970s and early 1980s also saw a sharp rise in unemployment, most notably amongst the young who often experienced very long periods out of work. In 1979, 57,000 under-25s were unemployed for over 12 months; by 1984, this figure had increased to 349,000 (Coffield *et al.* 1986). Under-18s were particularly badly affected: this group saw an 83 per cent increase in unemployment in the period 1979–84 (Harris 1989).

An obvious consequence of the limited employment opportunities facing the young was an increased reliance on state benefits and a shift into board and lodgings – a type of accommodation with cheap and easy access. The number of young people in this type of accommodation spiralled from 23,000 in 1982 to 85,000 in 1985 (*The Times*, 14.8.85). The need to institute cuts became evident as expenditure on this area of welfare rose alarmingly: even within the two years from December 1982 to December 1984, board and lodgings payments had more than doubled, from a total of £166m to £380m (*Hansard* (Commons), 20.11.85: 367). Similarly, the introduction of the SRR took place in the context of concerns related to marked increases in the Housing Benefit bill. Since 1987/8, Housing Benefit expenditure has increased more than sixfold, so leading to general attempts to curb costs (Wilcox 1997). For example, in January 1996, the Housing Benefit (General) Amendment Regulations 1995 came into effect, introducing the local reference rent regulations which essentially established a system whereby maximum Housing Benefit payments would be set as the equivalent of the average local market rent for that property type (*HA Weekly*, 24.11.95). Further cuts targeted the young, and the introduction of the SRR was rarely discussed without some reference to savings: in announcing the change, Peter Lilley – then Secretary of state for Social Security – claimed that the regulation would save an estimated £100m in its first year (*Independent*, 30.11.95).

Strategies to contain expenditure on private rental assistance for the young were also often justified by the need to prioritise, and target limited resources on those in greatest need. For example, the cuts to board and lodgings payments were accompanied by the assertion that the increases in payments had gone beyond what the Minister for Social Security and the Disabled called 'sensible social priorities' (*The Times*, 22.3.85). It was claimed that the abolition of the householder status and its replacement with an age distinction 'enabled the Government to concentrate more resources on older people – including pensioners and disabled people living in other people's households' (Secretary of State for Social Services 1985a: para 3:13). Similarly, when Kenneth Clarke, then Chancellor of the Exchequer, announced the SRR in his Budget speech of November 1995, he quickly justified the move by stating that 'It is by restricting spending in these areas that we can protect people in greatest need and stand by our pledges on pensions and child benefit' (*Independent Budget Special*, 29.11.95). This strategy of stressing the greater need of other groups to justify cuts in the entitlement of young people has often, in the case of housing in particular, been accompanied by associated rhetoric that downplayed the need of young people to receive assistance. Indeed, from the mid-1980s, the most consistent theme running through debate on young people's need for help with private rents has been assumptions on the way in which young people abuse their entitlement to benefit, principally by moving to properties they would not otherwise be able to afford.

Perhaps the most obvious case in which the supposed behaviour of young people was used to justify a reduction in their rental assistance was the change to board and lodgings payments. The summer of 1985 was beset with scandal attached to the belief that the rapid rise in payments could be explained by young people using the benefit to fund their living in hotels in holiday resorts: the so-called 'Costa del Dole' scam. According to the newspapers, hoteliers quickly caught on to the trend, and began encouraging young people to leave home and enjoy 'dole by the sea' (*The Times*, 22.3.85). MPs debating the issue in the House called up examples of their own: there was reference to 'schoolgirl daughters . . . paid for by the DSS' who had 'left home to live with their boyfriends in Morecambe' (*Hansard* (Commons), 20.11.85: 377). Generally it was claimed that 'young people ought not to be able to leave home at the drop of a hat and pick up large sums of taxpayers' money' (ibid.: 372). Critics pointed out that there was no evidence to suggest that young people's housing decisions were being led by the availability of the payments: for example, MP Tam Dalyell asserted that policy should not be made on the basis of newspaper anecdotes. However, the board and lodgings time restrictions directly responded to the media stories by being applied with particular stringency in seaside resorts, where the maximum time limit for payments was two weeks.

By contrast to the 'Costa del Dole' issue, the abolition of the householder/non-householder test in favour of an age distinction did not take place in the context of any exuberant claims for the behaviour of young people. Indeed, government statements down-played the shift to an age-related policy by claiming that it made sense to replace the unwieldy and administratively complex house-holder test by a much simpler proxy. Since most under-25s lived at home with their parents it could be assumed fair to grant them the restricted non-householder benefit level automatically. Most young people had left home by their mid-20s, so a 'householder' benefit level for all over-25s could similarly be assumed to be reason-able. However, even before new benefit rates were implemented, the age differential was attacked. The Social Security Advisory Com-mittee (SSAC) contended that there was 'no justification' for using age as a proxy for householder status, and that the new regulation was 'so simple as to be crude'. It was claimed that 58 per cent of 24-year-olds were householders or joint householders, so making a distinction at the age of 25 did not take 'social realities' into account. Furthermore, the SSAC criticised one of the underlying themes of the change: the implication that families should be responsible for accommodating young people until the age of 25 (Barclay 1985). Despite these and continuing criticisms, age-discriminatory help with rental costs was retained, and has been underlined with par-ticular force with the introduction of the SRR.

Debate surrounding the introduction of the SRR was redolent with the rhetoric of past battles on the issue of housing help for the young. A whole flurry of familiar assumptions was presented by Peter Lilley in justification for the new regulation: it would remove any inducement to leave the parental home; it would en-courage young people to live in a similar style of accommodation as their working peers; and – in a surprise revisit to an earlier and still unproven contention – it would 'reduce the attraction of moving to seaside resorts' (*Independent*, 30.11.95). In response, the SRR was reviewed and attacked with particular cogency by Baroness Hollis in the House of Lords:

> Why have the Government targeted the under 25s? It is in the belief that young people under 25 can and should live at

home. The Government believe that they do not do so because they are enticed into their own luxury accommodation through the generosity of Housing Benefit. The argument goes: cut Housing Benefit, get young people to shop around for cheaper accommodation – or better still, go home – the DSS bill will at a stroke be cut by £65 million and one will simultaneously strengthen family life. Every point of that analysis . . . is false.

(*Hansard* (Lords), 14.5.96: col. 438)

In further support of this argument, Earl Russell contended that an extended stay in the parental home was 'an unnecessary indignity': people of 24 'are not children and their parents do not want to treat them as children' (ibid. col.: 435). Again, critics pointed to a lack of research indicating that young people's housing behaviour was being distorted by the availability of benefit. Reference was made to a report that had been funded by the DSS itself, that found young people were unlikely to be induced to leave home by the availability of Housing Benefit (Kemp *et al.* 1994). Further research, funded by the then Department of the Environment, also came to the same conclusion and noted that young people were less likely to claim Housing Benefit than other groups, even when entitled to do so (H. Green *et al.* 1996: 113). The government itself admitted that, for the most part, young people 'live in modest accommodation, such as bedsits and rooms in shared flats and houses', but still appeared to hold the view that under-25s on Housing Benefit somehow had different expectations. The SRR was necessary to reinforce 'normal' behaviour (*Hansard* (Lords), 14.5.96: col. 444).

Thus, rationales for the implementation of restricted housing assistance for young people have to a large degree rested on the need to reduce welfare expenditure and target those groups in greatest need. A supporting theme has been young people's supposed abuse of help with housing costs, and the way in which the availability of help has distorted young people's housing behaviour. However, these assumptions are largely untested and the next section explores the difficulties relating to any assessment of the impact on housing decisions of assistance with rental costs. The next section also examines young people's uses of the private rented sector in the light of Housing Benefit restrictions, focusing particularly on the operation of the SRR.

ASSESSING THE IMPACT OF HOUSING BENEFIT RESTRICTIONS

Attempting to assess the impact of Housing Benefit restrictions on young people in the PRS is a complex process. This chapter has shown that a great deal of policy relating to assistance with private rental costs rests on the belief that young people take the availability of benefit into account when making a housing decision such as leaving the parental home or moving within the PRS. Indeed, it is supposed that the benefit recipient has such an accurate and full appreciation of the workings of the benefit system that their behaviour can be manipulated by changes in regulation. However, the government's own advisers call into question this somewhat unrealistic assumption. For example, in criticising the Conservative government's decision to press ahead with an under-60s SRR, the Social Security Advisory Committee (SSAC) argued that no clear conclusions could be drawn from the operation of the under-25s regulations: 'there is sufficient uncertainty about this to make it unsafe to proceed with the current proposals' (Social Security Advisory Committee 1997: 13).

Empirical research indicates that benefit recipients do not act as economic agents with perfect knowledge of the benefit system (for example, Cordon and Craig 1991; Ford *et al.* 1995a). Indeed, it is unwise to make any a priori judgements either about understanding of the benefit or knowledge that the benefit is available. DSS-funded research on the effect of benefits on housing decisions included qualitative interviews with Housing Benefit recipients and people in receipt of Income Support Mortgage Interest (ISMI) payments. Exploratory interviews also took place with a small sample of young people who were in households where the head of household was in receipt of ISMI. The sample was by no means representative, and further research needs to be completed in this area to draw more concrete conclusions. However, the study found that the young people who were interviewed had a limited understanding of Housing Benefit, and indeed comparing this group with the Housing Benefit recipients indicated that knowledge of the benefit tended to be acquired after a move was first taken. It was concluded that it cannot be assumed that young people living in the parental home are necessarily aware of the availability of help with housing costs. Furthermore, although tenants already in receipt of Housing Benefit had a relatively sophisticated understanding of the benefit system, there was still a degree of risk thought to be attached to moving tenancy whilst on benefit since it could not be guaranteed that all the rent at the new property would be covered by a reapplication for Housing Benefit (Kemp *et al.* 1994). A more recent study of young people's experience of the SRR came to similar conclusions: that it was difficult to 'second guess' the level of benefit that would be paid, and in these circumstances, minimising the risk of being left with a substantial shortfall was thought to be the best strategy (Kemp and Rugg 1998). Housing Benefit recipients in both studies, therefore, applied a great deal of caution to their housing choices: rents were at or below levels that were thought to be reasonable in terms of the likelihood of getting the full cost covered by Housing Benefit.

Research has indicated that a further factor needs to be taken into account in assessing the impact of Housing Benefit changes: the supply-side response of the private rented sector. Restrictive Housing Benefit regulations have been implemented in the belief that landlords will be eager to meet moderated demand with an appropriate accommodation supply. Even as late as 1996, the Conservative government was claiming – in defence of the SRR – that 'The rental market is flexible . . . We believe it will respond to changes in demand arising from the new Housing Benefit rules' (*Hansard*, 6.12.96: col. 794w). This claim was made in the context of a long series of well-publicised studies – some funded by the government itself – that demonstrated the unwillingness of landlords to deal with Housing Benefit recipients (for example, Kemp and Rhodes 1994a; Bevan *et al.* 1995; Crook *et al.* 1995; Rugg 1996). Since the introduction of the reference rent in 1996, landlord representative groups have been vociferous in protesting against having to accept lower Housing Benefit payments. For example, the National Federation of Residential Landlords baldly stated 'the Department of Social Security could be deluding itself that sufficient supply will continue to be forthcoming under the new scheme for housing benefit which they envisage' (*Residential Renting* 1997: 21). More recent studies are now moving beyond logging the reluctance of landlords to respond to Housing Benefit changes, and indicate that greater subtlety is needed. In particular, it has been demonstrated that variety in types of rental market will dictate a range of different supply-side responses. For example, landlords in a given city are more unlikely to let to benefit recipients if there is competing demand for accommodation from students or holiday-makers. Where competition for rented accommodation is low, land-lords are more likely to continue letting to young people (Kemp and Rugg 1998).

It is this aspect of Housing Benefit impact assessment that has proved to be by far the most important in addressing the conse-quences of the SRR. Recent research on the impact of the SRR – based on 56 interviews with young people on housing benefit, completed in six case study areas – has questioned the assumption that the SRR would force young people on Housing Benefit out of independent, self-contained accommodation and into shared property. The research found that young people already sought to live in this sort of accommodation. Almost all the young people in the sample were pragmatic enough to conclude that even if their preference might be self-contained accommodation, their incomes – largely based on low-paid, erratic or part-time work – would only cover the cost of sharing. Even if this was not the case, many of those interviewed actually expressed a preference for sharing, so long as they were sharing with people they knew (Kemp and Rugg 1998). Thus the only behaviour that was being affected by the benefit change was that of landlords, who were showing a growing un-willingness to let to young people. This move had been anticipated before the regulations were implemented (Rugg 1997), and has been confirmed by a number of reports produced by voluntary sector agencies that aim to place young people in housing need in properties in the PRS (Cutts 1997; Holmström 1997; Chugg 1998).

In these circumstances, young people's use of the PRS as transi-tional housing is likely to become restricted and problematic. For most young people, the primary transitional use of the PRS will be in the event of a first move from the parental home. Jones (1995b) demonstrated that, of the 35 per cent of 19-year-olds taking the first move out of the parental home, 25 per cent move into private rented housing. A great deal of research has demon-strated that the first move from the parental home is rarely smooth or linear, and that young people are likely to return if attempts to set up independent households run into difficulties and fail. As Coles *et al.* (this volume) have indicated, one response to problems in entering the housing market has been for young people simply to remain in the parental home for longer time periods. An alternative response may be the transitional period becomes more fractured and more closely associated with the incidence of employment and unemployment. Thus, as young people feel able to move out when they have work, loss of that work will also mean a breakdown of tenancy as young people will be unable to meet over a long period the shortfall between the asking rent and the SRR. It may also be the case that the inability to use the PRS as a transition period could lead to a higher incidence of failure in the 'lifetime' tenures. Future trends may see young people entering into owner occupation or social housing straight from the parental home without an extended experience of independent housing, and so may lack general householder skills, which could lead to difficulties, for example, with budgeting (A.E. Green *et al.* 1997).

The SRR also has an impact on young people's ability to use the PRS as residual housing. As with transitional housing, the PRS will not be amenable for use as a 'safety net' tenure if supply is restricted because of young people's reliance on benefit. In addition, a reliance on private renting as a long-term housing option means that issues relating to security of tenure and quality of accommodation become much more important. Without access to funds for deposit payments and rent in advance, young people may not be able to secure properties of sufficient quality and security to act as long-term housing. Where rental options are limited, young people are more likely to find themselves in lower-standard HMOs, sharing with strangers in a housing situation they are unlikely to want to sustain (Rugg and Kemp 1998). In these circumstances, where the rental market is not able or willing to respond to need amongst this group, then homelessness becomes a more likely outcome (Greve with Currie 1991).

CONCLUSION

This chapter has discussed the ways in which young people use private renting, and policy changes that have been based on claims of abuse by young people of their entitlement to help with rental costs. Successive governments have implemented increasingly stringent restrictions on young people's assistance with rental costs. Although much of this policy has been driven by the desire to curb welfare expenditure, its implementation has also been justified by the use of rhetoric that stresses the way in which benefit operates to distort young people's behaviour in the rental market. None of these changes have been based on evidence demonstrating that benefit does indeed have the claimed effect: on the contrary, research has shown that young people – obviously disadvantaged by their housing and welfare inexperience – if anything act cautiously in the rental market, and seek to reduce the risk of incurring insupportable housing costs by choosing properties at the cheapest end of the market.

As a consequence of the benefit changes, young people's uses of the PRS have been restricted. It is possible to claim that transitional uses may become more fractured as young people moving in and out of work find themselves unable to sustain tenancies. Alternatively, young people may opt out of transitional housing altogether, and take their first step out of the parental home straight into a lifetime tenure. Private renting as a residual tenure is also made difficult: young renters are already on the margins of acceptability with respect to landlords' letting preferences, and the introduction of the SRR has proved in many cases to be one disincentive too many.

Chapter 5

Students and housing

A testing time?

David Rhodes

Full-time students now comprise a large, and still increasing, group of people. They are a section of the population that form a specific key demand group for housing, having relatively clearly defined requirements which set them apart from most other people of a similar age. Despite this being the case, however, there has been little examination of how students' housing needs are met, how local housing markets respond to their demand, and the nature of the interaction between full-time students and other competing demand groups for housing. This chapter therefore explores issues pertaining to the housing situations of full-time students who are in attendance at establishments of higher education.

As a result of the limited systematic information available on students' housing markets, a relatively speculative approach has been taken in this chapter. Much of the evidence which is available is *ad hoc* and localised in focus, and little of it is up to date. In the absence of any large-scale and systematic information, therefore, the aim of this chapter is to discuss in a general way some of the issues surrounding student housing markets at the current time. Although the chapter is speculative, it comprises an exploration of some of the relevant literature as a precursor to a forthcoming national study of student housing markets, which has been funded by the Joseph Rowntree Foundation.

A GENERAL PICTURE OF STUDENT HOUSING

As noted in Coles *et al.* (this volume), students in full-time education have specific housing requirements. For the duration of their studies the majority of them have housing needs which are flexible in character. In particular, a key feature is the temporary nature of their demand for accommodation away from their parental home and in the locality of their university or college of higher education. Some full-time students will of course continue to live in the parental home, perhaps because of the establishment's proximity, or because it is made possible by the structure of their chosen course of study. Such students, however, generally represent a small minority of the total.

For most students, separate term-time accommodation away from the parental home is either necessary or desirable. This convention is particularly the case in recent times, with the incidence of students living at home during term-time having shown a marked decrease. During the 1959/60 academic year at the University of Edinburgh, for example, 36 per cent of students were studying in the parental home, but by 1988/9 this figure had fallen to just over 8 per cent (Nicholson and Wasoff 1989). More recent evidence on students at the University of York shows that during the 1994/5 academic year, 6 per cent were living at home with their parents during term-time (Rugg *et al.* 1995). A small minority of students might be owner occupiers, Nicholson and Wasoff reporting that just over 11 per cent of students at the University of Edinburgh in 1988/9 were of this type. Such people might be either mature entrants or temporary owners during their time of study, the latter possibly letting spare rooms to other students.

The vast majority of full-time students live, at least during their term-times, in the private rented sector (PRS), although there will inevitably be differences in the extent to which this occurs. For example, some evidence indicates that as many as one-third of Scottish students study within the parental home setting (Kemp and Willington 1995), although the example of Edinburgh University students shows that this proportion is by no means uniform. Other evidence indicates that there is some variation in the extent to which students use the PRS according to their type of educational institution, but even so the overwhelming proportion of students of the different types of establishment live in private rented accommodation of one sort or another (Rugg *et al.* 1995).

THE PRIVATE RENTED SECTOR

The nature of the private rented sector is highly differentiated in terms of both the supply of and demand for lettings. The tenure can be defined in terms of its supply-side, or ownership, characteristics. These comprise a variety of arrangements including private individuals, partnerships, companies, and a range of institutions (such as the Church, and the Ministry of Defence). Recent research shows that most PRS landlords are private individuals, and most have only a few (less than ten) lettings (Crook and Kemp 1996). Private landlords can be further categorised into those which operate as full-time businesses, and those that are sideline landlords for which letting is a part-time activity (Bevan *et al.* 1995). The importance of this distinction lies in the motivations and attitudes to letting which may be associated with different types of landlord, and which may ultimately impact on the opportunities for different types of demand group to gain access to the PRS (see for example, Bevan *et al.* 1995; Thomas *et al.* 1995). For example, Bevan *et al.* identified a group of sideline landlords which operated in a very informal manner. They were frequently only letting temporarily to help out a family member or a friend, and often did not think of themselves as landlords at all.

On the demand side of the PRS, four key groups have been identified (Bovaird *et al.* 1985). First, there is a slowly shrinking group of mostly elderly people who have always lived in the sector. Second, there are young and mobile households which require the relative flexibility and ease of access offered by the sector. Third, there are households living in lettings which are connected with employment or which have some other form of institutional link. Fourth, the sector performs a 'residual role' for low income households that have difficulty accessing owner occupation or social rented housing.

So far as students are concerned, the third demand-side category represents an important distinction, as it relates to lettings which are accessible to the public (the open market private rented sector) and those which are not. Many of the lettings which are inaccessible to the public are linked with employment ('tied lettings'), and particularly in the agricultural sector, such as farm-workers' cottages. However, many are institutionally owned, and this includes higher education establishments that are providing accommodation for the sole use of their own students – in halls of residence and other university-owned accommodation. Students therefore occupy a relatively privileged position, as in addition to housing in the open market PRS they have the potential to access accommodation provided by their institution. This situation has no reciprocal advantage for most other competing groups for the open market PRS. Usually, however, there are limitations imposed on access to accommodation provided by educational establishments, priority often being given to first-year students for example. For most students, therefore, the open market private rented sector represents their key source of housing for at least a portion of their time of study. In seeking to live in the open market private rented sector, full-time students will primarily be in competition with other young and mobile households, and also low income households which have difficulty entering into home ownership or social rented housing.

The open market PRS comprises the largest proportion of private lettings, the 1991 census showing that slightly under four-fifths of English households were living in this part of the sector. Amongst these households, approximately half were renting their letting furnished, and about half were renting unfurnished accommodation. Evidence indicates that the furnished subsector of the open market PRS invariably caters for students. The study at the University of Edinburgh shows that slightly more than three-quarters of the total number of students had term-time addresses in the private rented sector. Over half of these (39 per cent of the total) were living in the open market part of the sector, and virtually all of these were renting furnished accommodation. The remainder of the Edinburgh students were living in a variety of accommodation types owned by the university, and were therefore occupying PRS lettings which were inaccessible to the public. The situation at the University of York, reported in Rugg et al. (1995), was equally marked, with 54 per cent of students living in accommodation owned by the university and 31 per cent in the open market private rented sector.

RECENT DEVELOPMENTS

The current reliance of students on the open market PRS is the result of an historical development which has its roots in the early 1960s. At this time there was cross-party agreement on the need for an expansion of higher education as a matter of economic necessity, and as a basic individual right. What became known as the Robbins

Report (Committee on Higher Education 1963) made the point that expansion of university-provided accommodation would be necessary to facilitate the increased number of students. The Report considered it unrealistic to expect more than one-third of students to live either at home or in private rented lodgings, and that universities would therefore need to provide an increased amount of accommodation.

Student numbers have multiplied dramatically since the Robbins Report. Between 1962/3 and 1967/8 the number of students increased from 217,000 to 370,000, and then reached 524,000 in 1980/1 (Jones and Wallace 1992). The National Committee of Inquiry into Higher Education (1997) stated that this figure had grown to 1.6 million by 1995/6. Even by the end of the 1960s, however, universities had been unable to expand their provision of accommodation in line with the rise in student numbers. The reasons for this were in part due to the increased costs of building and high interest rates, but also because of the restrictions placed on grants to universities (Morgan and McDowell 1979). More recently, and although the previous government's target for one-third of all young people to enter full-time education by the end of the century has already been met, the Dearing Report (as the National Committee Inquiry into Higher Education Report is known) predicts that demand for higher education will still continue to increase from people of all ages. Despite the inevitable impact on local areas of increased student numbers, the housing implications were not addressed in the Report.

Over the same time-scale, the private rented sector has undergone considerable decline. In 1960 there were 4.6 million dwellings in the private rented sector, which represented 32 per cent of the total housing stock in England and Wales, and by the mid-1970s the sector had reduced to 2.9 million dwellings, or 16 per cent of the total stock (Kemp 1988). Since then, the private rented sector has declined in size even further, comprising 10.3 per cent of all English dwellings in 1996, 8.5 per cent of all Welsh dwellings in 1996, and 6.9 per cent of all Scottish dwellings in 1995 (Wilcox 1997).

Another change which may have had an impact on students' housing situations is the staged removal of their entitlement to benefits. During the 1986/7 academic year, students lost entitlement to income support and unemployment benefit during the short vacations, and those living in university-owned accommodation became no longer eligible for Housing Benefit. Since the summer of 1987, students living in the PRS were no longer eligible for Housing Benefit over the summer vacation. Except in certain excluded cases (lone parents, and those entitled to disability allowances), September 1990 saw student entitlement to benefits withdrawn completely, they now being ineligible for Housing Benefit all year round, and for income support during the summer vacation.

In addition to the benefit changes, maintenance grants were frozen by the Conservative government at 1990/1 levels allowing them to be eroded by inflation, although their real value since the introduction of grants in 1962 had fallen by about one-fifth by the end of the 1980s (DES 1988). Student loans were therefore introduced in 1990 as a measure to allow students to top up their grants. Although their sources of income have changed since the late 1980s and the early 1990s (with the introduction of loans and more students working part-time), the real value of students' incomes had on average risen by the 1995/6 academic year (Callender and Kempson 1996). A further development occurred in October 1998, from which time many students will be required to make a contribution towards their tuition costs. It is unclear how the payment of fees will impact on students' total incomes at the time of writing. There could, however, be a knock-on affect for local housing markets (and ultimately higher education establishments themselves), should the extra cost be reflected in new entrants choosing to study in areas with the lowest accommodation costs (which vary considerably and consume a large proportion of students' income, as is discussed below).

STUDENTS AND LOCAL HOUSING MARKETS

Governments in the past have had no clearly defined housing policy for full-time students (Brown 1992), and this is still the case despite the 1997 Dearing Report prediction for the number of students to continue increasing. Largely as a result of this lack of central guidance, the housing opportunities for students, and by implication those of other competing groups in areas containing universities and higher education colleges, will vary. Some of the factors likely to influence local housing markets include the extent of institutionally provided accommodation, total student numbers, the size of the local open market PRS, the characteristics of local landlords, the number and tenant type of other groups competing for the open market PRS, local rent levels, and the flow (or turnover) of lettings in the PRS. All these things will vary to some extent from one area to the next, and hence make it difficult to generalise about the 'typical' or 'traditional' student housing experience, as perhaps has been possible in the past.

The above studies in Edinburgh and York together show two things. First, that there is much use of the open market private rented sector by students; and second, that there is also variation from one area to the next in the extent to how heavily this part of the sector is relied on. As a result, students' housing experiences are far from uniform. This diversity is supported by other more anecdotal evidence, which indicates a far wider range of housing situations than is suggested by these two studies alone. The *Which University* guide (Allen 1994) is aimed at prospective students, and contains brief descriptions of the housing arrangements at individual institutions. At the University of Kent in Canterbury, for example, 52 per cent of its 6,000 students live in college, and all first year students who accept the offer of a place before a given date are guaranteed university accommodation. However, 'with swelling numbers increasing the pressure on housing, the advice is to get in there fast' (Allen 1994: 166). The guide also indicates that due to pressure on the PRS in the city, some students end up living several miles away in the surrounding towns. A contrasting picture is presented by the London Guildhall University. The university has 94 per cent of its 14,000 students living in the open market PRS, and 'No student is guaranteed accommodation, and details of what is available are not automatically forwarded to new students' (Allen 1994: 362). The guide goes on to indicate that the accommodation office at this university has lists of PRS accommodation, which includes hostels and bedsits, as well as shared houses and flats.

In the context of the recent changes to the private rented sector, and also to student numbers, it is unclear how local housing markets are responding at the present time. However, research conducted during the 1970s examined the situation in Brighton (McDowell 1978). McDowell notes that the expansion in student numbers in Brighton at that time had not been matched by a growth in institutionally provided accommodation, and that students in the area had been increasingly looking to live in the open market PRS. Some important supply-side issues were raised by this study, which suggest that students may have had a competitive advantage. First, it was apparent that students often had an advantage over other demand groups for larger accommodation as, by sharing housing, several students together were able to afford higher rents. Second, the size of a student household is flexible, and can more readily adjust to different property sizes than is the case with, for example, a family which is looking for somewhere to rent.

On the demand side, a crucial dimension for people looking to live in the open market private rented sector is the nature of private landlords' letting preferences. A representative survey of private landlords in England found that the most preferred type of tenant in terms of economic status, for both landlords and managing agents, was people in work (Crook and Kemp 1996). This finding accords with the results of other PRS surveys (for example, Kemp and Rhodes 1994a). Importantly, however, Crook and Kemp found that second to unemployed people, students were the least preferred type of tenant by both landlords (24 per cent) and managing agents (29 per cent). Students also fared poorly in terms of the most and least preferred household type, with only 7 per cent of all landlords most preferring young single people. Landlords and managing agents alike (38 per cent for both) least preferred letting to young single people more than any other household type.

These findings from national surveys, however, do not mean that at a local level landlords will always be able to operationalise their preferments, and in some cases they have been found to be letting to their least favoured tenant type (Kemp and Rhodes 1994b). Landlords will of course also be guided by the necessity to minimise voids (vacancies between tenancies), and may not be able to wait until they find their most preferred tenant type. The preferences of private landlords will also be related to the type of accommodation which they let, and which may be inappropriate for some tenant types. A study of houses in multiple occupation and board and lodgings in Glasgow (Kemp and Rhodes 1994b), for example, found that contrary to the national pattern, many landlords (27 per cent) most preferred to let to young single people.

The study by Rugg et al. (1995) also confirmed the point raised in the Brighton research, finding that many landlords had a preference for letting to students. The reason for this was because a higher total rent could be obtained from a household comprising several students than from other types of household which had a single income or which were reliant on benefits. The York study found that landlords were responding directly to the demand for accommodation from students, in buying houses for furnished letting in areas near to the city's higher education institutions. Such niche landlord activity has been found in other research on the PRS (Trickett 1995). An implication of this situation is that student demand in some areas for shared housing may push out families seeking larger accommodation. A different experience was evident in Liverpool, where private landlords did not appear to have specifically targeted student households. Rather, the increase in student numbers during the 1980s had complemented a reduction in demand for the PRS from the local population: 'students have moved in as Scousers have moved out' (Allen 1994: 341).

The extent to which full-time students are able to secure open market PRS accommodation will also depend on the size of this part of the sector, and the flow of lettings becoming available throughout the year. Table 5.1 shows selected areas containing

Table 5.1 Open market PRS stock and estimated annual flow of furnished lettings

Local authority area	Open market PRS stock (no.)	(% of all)	Annual flow of furnished lettings (no.)	(% of PRS stock)
Birmingham	24,754	6.6	7,520	30.4
Bristol	14,535	9.3	5,144	35.4
Cambridge	5,997	15.2	2,874	47.9
Kingston upon Hull	9,198	8.9	2,116	23.0
Leeds	18,822	6.7	6,604	35.1
Lincoln	2,737	8.0	1,015	37.1
Manchester	19,845	11.7	7,553	38.1
Newcastle upon Tyne	10,044	9.0	2,871	28.6
Nottingham	9,256	8.5	3,071	33.2
Oxford	7,008	16.0	2,483	35.4
Sheffield	12,773	6.0	4,354	34.1
York	3,703	8.8	1,498	40.4

Sources: 1991 census (own analysis). Material from Crown copyright records, made available through the Office of Population Censuses and Surveys and the ESRC Data Archive, has been used by permission of the Controller of HM Stationery Office.

Notes: Open market PRS stock figures are adjusted to account for the growth in the size of the sector since the census, and also to exclude dwellings unfit for human habitation. The annual flow has been calculated from the average length of residence in the furnished and unfurnished subsectors in different types of local authority area. Further details of the methods are contained in Rhodes and Bevan (1997). The census contains counts of households, which have been taken as a proxy for the stock of dwellings.

student populations, the relative size of the open market PRS, and the estimated annual flow (turnover) of furnished lettings. The table is based on an analysis of households contained in the 1991 census, and indicates considerable variation between different areas. The number of students in each area will of course also have an impact, and research to identify areas of high student demand – often from several institutions in an area – would provide valuable information on the way in which local housing markets are operating. In the absence of this information, however, the figures in the table suggest that other things being equal students may find it more difficult to secure open market accommodation in for example Newcastle upon Tyne, where the annual flows of furnished lettings are comparatively small, than they would in Cambridge, where the flow is much higher and the open market PRS as a proportion of the total stock is larger. The figures in the table do not, of course, take any account of variations in demand from students throughout the year, and which can result in large scarcity for students at the beginning of the academic year (for example, Hancock 1997).

In addition to differences in the size of open market PRS stock and annual flow of lettings, there are also large variations between local housing markets in average rent levels. Such variation is clearly important, as the amount of students' total income spent on paying the rent can be high. For example, Kemp and Rhodes (1994b) found in their 1992 study of the lower end of the PRS in Glasgow that students were on average paying 59 per cent of their income on rent.

As might be expected, rents are often much the highest in Greater London. To some extent this situation is reflected in the larger grants and maximum loans available to students living in the capital, although rents have been found to vary considerably within the area (Rhodes and Kemp 1998). Throughout the rest of the country a uniform and lower level of grant and loan is available to full-time students. However, average rents throughout the rest of England, Scotland and Wales vary considerably, as the following examples illustrate. The figures are based on the average open market PRS rent for two bedroom furnished terraced houses in the fourth quarter of 1997 in areas with significant student populations. This size of property might be shared by two or perhaps three students, depending on living arrangements, although the patterns identified hold for other sizes and types of property. In Nottingham the rent was £63 per week, in Leeds it was £65 per week, in Manchester it was £80 per week, in Glasgow it was £85 per week, in Cardiff it was £95 per week, in Cambridge it was £133 per week, in Brighton it was £135 per week, and in Aberdeen it was £166 per week (Rhodes and Kemp 1998).

Rent levels in institutionally provided accommodation also vary from place to place. For a self-catering single room in the 1996/7 academic year, for example, the average rent was £26.74 per week at the University of St Andrews, £33.46 per week at the University of Hull, £39.40 per week at the University of Bath, and £48 per week at Nottingham Trent University (NUS 1996). Despite what might at first glance appear to be preferential rent levels in accommodation provided by educational establishments, students may often find open market PRS accommodation more affordable. For example, the average amount of income spent on rent by students living in institutionally provided accommodation during 1996/97 was 63 per cent, compared with 52 per cent in the open market PRS (NUS 1996). The lower proportion of income spent on rent in the open market PRS is most likely due to students living in shared housing. Research in Scotland suggests that increased occupancy rates amongst students in the open market PRS is one way in which they deal with the high cost of accommodation relative to their incomes (Kemp and Willington 1995). Students may also prefer to live in the open market PRS because of the choice it offers them to make savings in other areas, such as on heating, lighting and in some instances meals, which can be inclusive in halls of residence rents. It is possible that the generally higher proportion of income spent on rent in institutionally provided accommodation may be acting as a spur for an increasing number of students to seek accommodation in the open market PRS. However, there is no evidence to confirm the extent to which this process might be occurring.

The nature of the interaction between institutionally provided accommodation and the open market PRS is further complicated by recent changes to the Housing Benefit system (see Rugg, this volume). The Housing Act (1996) introduced Local Reference Rents for new Housing Benefit determinations. This regulation sets the maximum Housing Benefit payable to the average (mid point in the range excluding extreme values) of all non-Housing Benefit open market rents for similar sized property in the locality. Any shortfall between the Housing Benefit paid and the rent charged will have to be met by the recipient, or they will have to find cheaper accommodation, or they may be able to negotiate a lower rent level with the landlord. It is not clear how landlords are responding to this new regulation, but clearly one outcome is for the competitive balance to be tipped in students' favour relative to Housing Benefit tenants.

A further modification to the Housing Benefit system was the introduction in October 1996 of the Single Room Rent for claimants aged under 25. This regulation means that the maximum rent assistance available to single people aged under 25 is set to the mid point in the locality for all single rooms with shared use of facilities. The regulation applies whether the claimant lives in a single room in a shared house or not. Once again, it is unclear what sort of impact at a local level this regulation is having on the housing opportunities for students as well as other competing groups. One outcome might be, for example, that fewer single people are leaving the parental home to live independently, in which case there might be an increased supply of single rooms in shared housing for students. Alternatively, more single people may be looking to live in shared housing than might otherwise have been the case, and which could increase the supply of self-contained accommodation for students. A further alternative outcome might be that some landlords who catered for the Housing Benefit market might be withdrawing from letting completely. What will almost certainly be the case, however, is that different local markets will be responding to the new Housing Benefit regulations in different ways. For example, Kemp and Rugg (1998) found in one of their case study areas that despite the introduction of the single room rent, non-students were finding it easier to find shared accommodation because of an increased take-up by students of recently provided accommodation by the local universities.

The Edinburgh study noted that some landlords may prefer letting to students because of the regular and predictable vacancies each year, and which provide an opportunity for increasing rent levels. However, the increasingly widespread use of assured short-hold tenancies since the Edinburgh study, by which landlords can be sure of repossession after a minimum period of six months, may have served to negate that type of advantage, possibly placing students and other types of tenant on a more level playing field. In 1996/7, for example, 47 per cent of all PRS lettings, which was by far the largest single proportion, were assured shorthold tenancies (H. Green et al. 1998). This proportion represents a rapid increase, the figure in 1990 being just 8 per cent. In the absence of research evidence, however, it is unclear what sort of impact this increased usage of assured shorthold tenancies is having on the open market PRS in student areas.

There is evidence that some universities, and also private investors, have recently begun to invest in quality student accommodation, as it is increasingly seen as being important in attracting conferences during the student vacations. The likely impact on local housing markets depends very much on term-time rent levels, however, as reports indicate that the quality of the accommodation frequently puts the costs beyond most students (Spittles 1997).

CONCLUSIONS

This chapter has discussed some of the issues which are of relevance to student housing markets. As a result of a lack of hard evidence, and also because of recent changes which may impact on housing opportunities for students, it is unclear what might be happening at a local level. New research on students living in the open market PRS would provide a valuable contribution to the understanding of how local housing markets operate for both students and other competing groups, which need to be considered simultaneously, as one competing group's gain is another's loss.

Examination of the available evidence suggests that students may often have a competitive advantage over several other competing groups for the open market PRS. Students can easily form households of varying sizes to suit the accommodation available, and in doing so may often be in a position to afford rent levels that single-income households and benefit-dependent households cannot. As the York study showed, many private landlords in the city have in fact been responding to the higher returns available from letting to students. The recent changes to the Housing Benefit system have perhaps also tipped the competitive balance further in favour of students, whose overall income in recent years has on average increased. Furthermore, many full-time students will have access to institutionally provided accommodation – which other competing groups do not – although the extent of this varies widely.

It is difficult, however, to be conclusive about how individual student housing markets are operating at the current time, as a range of localised factors will impact at a local level. These include the size of the student population, the characteristics of local landlords, the size and type of other competing groups, the existence of formal relationships between universities and local landlords, the extent of institutionally provided accommodation, relative rent levels between the open market PRS and institutionally provided student accommodation, and the absolute size of the open market PRS and the annual flow of lettings becoming available.

Flexibility is often considered to be a key characteristic of the open market private rented sector, but this chapter has indicated that niche markets can operate at a local level, thereby suggesting a degree of rigidity. Little is known about this type of market behaviour, however, particularly in the context of the recent changes to the Housing Benefit system and the increasing numbers of students.

In addition to the lack of information in areas with well-established institutions of higher education, it is unclear what is happening to the open market PRS in cities where more recent development has taken place: for example, in the city of Lincoln which saw the opening of its new university in September 1996. The Dearing Report has predicted that student numbers would continue to increase, and yet gave no consideration to the need for additional student housing. It also reiterated the commitment to adult learning, but made no acknowledgement of the housing needs of students with families. The Report indicated that during 1995/6, 58 per cent of those in full-time education were mature students. In this context, the future may see an increase in the proportion of students who are owner occupiers, either buying somewhere to live near their university or, perhaps more likely, studying at institutions in their own locality. It also remains to be seen whether the introduction of tuition fees in October 1998 will have an impact on student housing markets, if the extra expenditure leads students to opt for courses in areas with low accommodation costs.

Chapter 6

'I thought it would be easier'

The early housing careers of young people leaving care

Nina Biehal and Jim Wade

Each year approximately 8,000 young people leave the care of local authorities and, if unable to return to their families, seek a place for themselves as young adults in the community. Concern at the vulnerability of young people leaving care has grown from the mid-1970s. Despite those looked after constituting less than 1 per cent of their age group, evidence from a range of studies and reports has persistently placed care leavers amongst the most disadvantaged. These concerns have rested upon the early age at which young people were expected to assume adult responsibilities and their lack of preparedness for the task (Stein and Carey 1986); the failure of the majority to attain qualifications at the end of their schooling and, in consequence, for large numbers to be unemployed once they have left care (Garnett 1992; Broad 1994; Biehal *et al.* 1995); and the tendency for those with a background in care to be over-represented amongst the young homeless (Randall 1989; Strathdee and Johnson 1994) and the prison population (National Children's Bureau 1992).

However, it is also the case that those who leave care aged 16 or over to live independently represent only a small proportion of the looked-after population. Young people may be looked after for a diverse range of reasons, most commonly to provide temporary relief to families under stress, and the majority return to their families after a short stay (Department of Health 1997). For those who remain during their teenage years, the local authority has a responsibility to help prepare them for the time when they will cease to be looked after and to support them through that transition, wherever possible in partnership with their families. While looked after, the quality of experience for young people has been shown to be variable. Although many young people have valued the experience of being looked after and felt it has helped them, for some it has tended to compound their difficulties. For those looked after longer, their careers have often been marked by further movement and disruption, by a tendency for links with family and community to weaken and, in consequence, for them to experience some identity confusion (Millham *et al.* 1986; Stein and Carey 1986). These feelings could be particularly acute for black young people brought up in a predominantly 'white' care context (First Key 1987).

Our discussion of young people's transitions from substitute care will draw upon the findings of a longitudinal study of the processes associated with this transition. Conducted soon after the implementation of the Children Act 1989, the study investigated the impact of differing leaving care schemes and approaches to the delivery of leaving care services in three local authorities. By means of a survey and follow-up interview sample it charted the experience of transition for young people over their first 18–24 months of independent living in the community and explored the support made available to them from carers, social workers and leaving care schemes (Biehal *et al.* 1992, 1995).

THE CHILDREN ACT 1989

The Children Act involved a major rewriting of both public and private law for children and families. Although subsequently there has been considerable debate about the degree to which it stood apart from or was consonant with other social policies introduced in the Thatcher era (Packman and Jordan 1991; Parton 1991), it was broadly welcomed as a positive set of measures. The main leaving care provisions were enshrined in Section 24 of the Act and its associated guidance (Department of Health 1991; Stein 1991). Local authorities were given a duty to prepare young people for the time when they will cease to be looked after. Guidance suggested that, in addition to equipping young people with the practical skills needed for self-reliance, preparation should focus on building self-esteem and an ability to build and maintain relationships. However, recent studies have suggested that, despite these provisions, the degree to which preparation is adequately planned and structured over time remains variable (Biehal *et al.* 1995; Clayden and Stein 1996).

In relation to aftercare support, local authorities have a duty to advise and befriend young people looked after to the age of 16 or beyond until they reach 21. Although the amount and range of this support is discretionary, guidance suggested that it could include someone to befriend the young person and help with education, training and housing. Local authorities are also empowered to provide financial assistance in cash or kind to assist in any of the above areas. One weakness in relation to the discretionary nature of these financial powers is that, certainly in the early years of the Act's implementation, it did little to remedy the regional disparities in the kinds of support young people could expect. At one end of the spectrum, some authorities used Section 24 funds imaginatively to fund specialist leaving care schemes to provide support and develop resource options, to offer leaving care grants to help furnish flats and to subsidise young people in education, training or low paid work while, at the other, some young people continued to receive little financial help at all (Lowe 1990; Garnett 1992; First Key 1992; Sone 1994). A recent inspection of leaving care procedures in nine local authorities suggested that, while the overall situation had improved, variations persisted and young people often lacked information about the financial help available (Social Services Inspectorate 1997). In addition, increasing restrictions on young people's access to social security and Housing Benefit has meant that social services departments have increasingly been required to use these funds to make up this shortfall in basic incomes (Biehal *et al.* 1995; Broad 1998).

Separate to the leaving care provisions, Section 20 (3) places a duty on local authorities to accommodate any 16- or 17-year-old 'in need' where to do otherwise would 'seriously prejudice' their health. If accommodated for more than 24 hours, young people become eligible for advice and support under Section 24. During the year 1994/5, 2,610 young people aged 16 or over were accommodated under this Section, the majority in foster or residential placements (Social Services Inspectorate 1997). The inspection mentioned above found these nine social service departments to be flexible in providing accommodation for this age group, but only two had formal agreements with their housing authorities that facilitated a reconciliation of 'serious prejudice' and 'in need' under the Children Act with the concept of 'vulnerability' in housing legislation and a framework for the joint assessment of homeless teenagers. This finding is consistent with other more specialist studies in this area (Kay 1994; McCluskey 1994). Kay found that few housing authorities accepted homeless 16–17 year olds as vulnerable by virtue of their age alone – an important plank of campaigns by homelessness agencies. Only one half of the authorities accepted leaving care as a sufficient 'other reason' in addition to age; and only one-quarter had changed their policies on vulnerability in the light of the Children Act. So although the duties and powers contained within the Children Act offer a framework for providing comprehensive services to young people leaving care and recognise the similar needs of homeless 16–17 year olds who have not been looked after, inconsistencies and variations in the development of those services persist.

TRANSITIONS FROM SUBSTITUTE CARE

Implementation of the Act has also taken place at a time of increasing financial restraint for local authorities and in the context of other social policies that have often had adverse effects on the lives of young people. The collapse of the youth labour market, the rapid growth of education and training, the decline of affordable housing, and welfare policies designed to deter young people from leaving home have created a new and more protracted context for the transition to adulthood. Transitions have tended to become more extended, less linear in shape, and the relationship between the different elements of transition – leaving home, acquiring financial independence, gaining adult citizenship and family formation – less closely associated (Jones and Wallace 1992; Coles 1995; Furlong and Cartmel 1997). Although there are more formal choices for young people, and transitions are experienced in more individualised ways, the risks involved are greater (Giddens 1991; Beck 1992), especially for those constrained to leave home before 18 and lacking consistent family support (Jones 1995b). This process of restructuring represented an important context for our investigation of young people's transitions from care in the 1990s.

Leaving care needs to be understood as a process, not a single discrete event, which involves young people in making a series of transitions – from their substitute homes to independent households, from school to further education or employment and, for some, the formation of their own families. For young people at large these elements of transition have tended to become more loosely connected and to extend over a number of years. In stark contrast, transitions for looked-after young people, who often lack reliable family support, tend to be both accelerated and compressed.

Looked-after young people are expected to move to independent living at a much earlier age than young people in the general population. In relation to our survey sample, 29 per cent moved to independence at the age of 16 and 60 per cent before the age of 18 (Biehal et al. 1992). This finding is consistent with earlier studies of care leavers (Stein and Carey 1986; Garnett 1992). The contrast with patterns for young people in the general population is quite striking. In the early 1980s the median age for leaving home was 22 for males and 20 for females (Jones 1987) and, although more recent evidence from the Scottish Young People's Survey points to a tendency for young people to first leave home at a younger age, this is still only the case for around one in ten of those aged under 18 (Jones 1995b).

Not only are young people expected to leave 'home' at an earlier age but the different strands of transition tend to be compressed into a short time period. For many young people in our study, moving from care to independent accommodation, attempting to find a niche in the youth labour market, setting up home with a partner and becoming a parent all occurred within 18–24 months of leaving care. For young people whose pasts have often been marked by instability, abuse and emotional distress, the assumption of full adult responsibilities in this way is likely to represent a severe test.

In particular the transition from school to work can prove difficult. Recent studies have shown that qualifications gained at 16 years of age represent the best single predictor of likely career routes (Banks et al. 1992; Roberts 1993) and, in this regard, looked-after young people are seriously disadvantaged. Surveys of care leavers have consistently found that between two-thirds and three-quarters leave school with no formal qualifications (Stein and Carey 1986; Garnett 1992; Biehal et al. 1995) and this is reflected in the pattern of their early post-school careers. Over a third of our survey sample and half of our interview sample were unemployed upon leaving care and two-thirds of those we interviewed had embarked on an 'insecure' career path, involving short-term casual work interspersed with episodes of training and lengthening bouts of unemployment. The importance of young people having a supportive base from which to launch their initial careers is reinforced by our finding that the majority of those who successfully start training or employment did so from the shelter of supported accommodation. These young people had either remained with foster carers or family or were placed in supported hostels or lodgings.

Not surprisingly, given these patterns, the majority of young people were being expected to manage on very low incomes. For young people often unable to rely on the important informal support that families can offer in such circumstances (Kirk *et al.* 1991; Jones 1995b), and in a context of increasing restrictions to social security benefits, many were dependent for their survival on additional financial assistance from social services. However, as we have indicated, the provision of such assistance is variable within and between authorities. Coping with poverty tended to stretch young people's life skills, increased their social isolation and, for some, threatened their ability to manage their homes.

Loneliness and isolation may also have been one factor associated with a tendency towards early family formation. Within 18–24 months of leaving care over one-third of the interview sample were living with partners, in some instances having 'adopted' their partners' families, and nearly half of the young women had become parents. All were aged 19 or under when their babies were born and, given that the average age of first time motherhood in the late 1980s was 26.5 years, the contrast with the general population is striking (Kiernan and Wicks 1990).

PROBLEMS ASSOCIATED WITH ACCELERATED TRANSITIONS

Transitions that are accelerated and, in many cases, compressed, can bring with them a concentration of difficulties which make it hard for many young people to manage independent living. If we focus solely on care leavers' entry into the housing market, their difficulties in this arena are evident in the high degree of mobility in their early housing careers and in high rates of homelessness.

Although some mobility is normal for this age group and may be positive, some care leavers make repeated moves for negative reasons. Within two years of leaving care, over half of the young people in our study had made two or more moves and a sixth had made five or more moves. Some moves were made when better accommodation became available, or when young people moved from intermediate households into independent tenancies. Some benefited from the support available in hostels or supported lodgings, while many of those in independent households managed reasonably well, especially if they received professional support. However, a number found it hard to budget, to cope with their new-found autonomy and isolation, and the lack of structure and day-to-day support at such an early age. Problems such as these led some young people to make repeated moves because they felt unable to manage tenancies of their own, found it hard to cope even in supported accommodation, or because they were fleeing violence or harassment. Instability in one area of young people's lives sometimes undermined positive developments in other areas, as moving often brought with it the disruption of further education, training or work, leading to a downward spiral.

For some the early transition to the housing market rapidly led to homelessness. Fifteen per cent of our survey sample had experienced homelessness within nine months of leaving care and over a fifth of those in our interview sample were homeless at some point within two years of leaving care, some of them on more than one occasion (Biehal et al. 1995). Many recent studies have found that between a fifth and a third of the young homeless have been in care at some point in their lives (Young Homelessness Group 1991; NCH 1993; Jones 1995; Smith et al. 1996; Markey 1998). Comparing homeless and non-homeless young people, Craig and colleagues found that those who were homeless were ten times more likely to have spent some time in statutory care during childhood (Craig et al. 1996). Research by Centrepoint's London hostels since the late 1980s has consistently found that around a third of their users had a care background (Randall 1988; Strathdee 1992; McCluskey 1994; Strathdee and Johnson 1994). By 1996 the situation appeared to have deteriorated, as Centrepoint reported that 40 per cent of its users had been in care and estimated that this was also a feature in the background of 28 per cent of the young homeless outside London (Nassor 1996).

Young people with a care background appear to be at higher risk of sleeping rough (Anderson et al. 1993; Strathdee and Johnson 1994; Markey 1998). Among those in our interview sample who became homeless, two-thirds slept rough or stayed in hostels for the homeless, while another study of homeless care leavers found that the vast majority had slept rough and had used emergency hostels (Kirby 1994). These findings suggest that young people with a care background are likely to have fewer support networks available to them in times of crisis.

For those who leave care at 16 or over, there is some indication of a relationship between an early entry to the housing market and patterns of homelessness. Our survey found a significant association between leaving care early, at only 16 or 17, and subsequent homelessness. This may be related to the manner in which younger care leavers left their final placements. All but one of those in our interview sample who left care as the result of a placement breakdown or other crisis did so before the age of 18. The crisis-driven manner in which they left precipitated them rapidly into independent living, often in emergency accommodation in bed and breakfast hotels, bedsits or board and lodgings, and most of these arrangements were short lived. Leaving care at only 16 or 17, particularly if this happens in an unplanned way, clearly increases the risk of homelessness for care leavers.

We also found a significant association between a high mobility while looked after and subsequent homelessness. For those who made numerous moves between residential and foster placements, preparation for leaving care may have been inadequate if they were not settled long enough to receive it. Young people who are looked after may also experience instability through persistently going missing from care placements. Recent research has shown that going missing from residential care is a serious problem for local authorities and that, among those young people who do go missing, a large minority do so repeatedly (Wade et al. 1998). British studies have found that many homeless young people with a care background have a history of running away from home or care, while North American research has identified running away as a precursor to adult homelessness (Simons and Whitbeck 1991; Kirby 1994; Craig et al. 1996; Markey 1998). Persistently going missing from care is associated with involvement in crime and substance misuse and with truancy and exclusion from school (Wade et al. 1998), all of which may make it particularly difficult for this group of young people subsequently to find employment and adapt to independent living at an early age. If young people are often missing from their care placements, then attempts to equip them with the kinds of practical and social skills they will need and to make effective plans for their futures may be impossible to achieve.

A consideration of the routes into homelessness for the young people in our interview sample who experienced it suggests that many were ill-prepared or unready for independent living. Some did not have the skills to sustain a tenancy or found it hard to cope with the loss of structure in their lives, which either led to their eviction or to their leaving their accommodation on impulse. Others had stayed temporarily with their families, but relationships had rapidly broken down. Other studies have also found that some care leavers become homeless after an initial return to the family home and that for those who return home, aftercare support is less consistent than for those moving to other accommodation (Kirby 1994; Social Services Inspectorate 1997).

It should therefore be clear that accelerated transitions – particularly where they occur in an unplanned, crisis-driven manner – bring with them a risk of homelessness at an early age. Those care leavers who become homeless are likely to have had unsettled care careers involving multiple placement moves or a history of going missing and, as a result, are ill-prepared for independence. In addition, homelessness among those with a care background must be understood in a wider policy context. Policy changes in the fields of housing and social security have reduced the availability of affordable housing for single people and increased the risk of poverty for unemployed young people, both of which have serious consequences for those without access to family support (McCluskey 1994). The provisions of the Children Act 1989 cannot, in isolation, sufficiently mitigate the effects of these wider policy changes which have made care leavers particularly vulnerable to homelessness.

ELEMENTS OF SUCCESSFUL TRANSITIONS

Understanding the risks associated with certain pathways out of care and the contexts in which more successful transitions occur can provide pointers to the elements of a good transition for care leavers. The most basic requirement of a good transition is that it should not occur too early. A cultural change is needed in the care system to counter the expectation on the part of managers, social workers, residential workers, foster carers and some young people that the move should be made at only 16 or 17 years of age, when young people are often not ready to cope with the demands of independent living. Early transitions are often a result of crisis moves out of care, which lead to hurried unplanned transitions to living situations which are unsupported and which rapidly break down. Attempts to prevent placement breakdown for teenagers would therefore also contribute to the achievement of more successful transitions.

The corollary of this is that transitions should be well planned and well supported. Careful preparation and detailed leaving care planning were important features of successful transitions in our study. Preparation that encouraged the development of informal support networks and plans which delineated the sources of support that would be available to young people were particularly valuable. For young people often lacking consistent family support, continuing care by social workers and carers is likely to be important as they attempt to find their feet in the adult world. However, a consistent finding of research in this area has been a tendency for planned support to fall away soon after legal discharge (Stein and Carey 1986; Biehal et al. 1992; Garnett 1992). Follow-up support by residential staff was extremely rare in our study, and that provided by foster carers declined once young people had moved on. A similar pattern was also apparent for social workers. Although two-fifths were still in touch at the end of the study, in most instances contact depended on young people approaching their worker if they needed help. If the aim is to ensure continuity of support for young people through a difficult set of transitions, then greater recognition and funding needs to be given to this continuing care role.

The availability of a range of accommodation options to meet differing needs can also contribute to good transitions. Looked-after young people do not form a homogeneous group: their past experiences and level of preparedness for moving on are likely to differ markedly. Many young people in our study who lacked the skills for independent living valued the intensive support available in trainer flats, hostels and supported lodgings. 'Floating support' schemes had advantages for those wanting lower levels of support. These forms of supported accommodation were an important resource for young people in our study.

For those ready and willing to try their own flats a supply of good quality permanent tenancies is needed. Securing a permanent tenancy at an early stage can provide valuable stability for those ready to cope with independent living. However, we found that the momentum of the planning process often played a part in determining the age at which young people moved to independence, since the time of moving on was governed by the time at which the offer of a tenancy was made. This was sometimes sooner than expected, leading to a hurried move, often before the young person was ready to take responsibility for an independent household. Closer co-operation between housing providers, social services and young people regarding the timing of offers of tenancies might reduce the risk of tenancies breaking down at an early stage.

Joint working of this kind would be in keeping with the Children Act 1989, which expects local authorities to adopt a corporate approach, so that their strategic planning for children's services, housing and community care addresses the housing needs of care leavers. The Code of Guidance to the Housing Act 1996 describes care leavers as one of the most vulnerable groups of young people and recommends that a joint assessment of their housing needs should be carried out by housing and social services departments as part of individual leaving care planning. This involvement of housing authorities in leaving care arrangements represents an important policy change (Brody 1996).

However local authorities organise their leaving care services, the development of an appropriate range of accommodation options represents a time-consuming and specialist function and one that may best be undertaken by a specialist leaving care scheme. Such a scheme requires an authority-wide overview of resources and formal partnerships with housing providers – statutory, voluntary and private. The development of joint initiatives also requires considerable investment by social services. The three authorities in our study, to varying degrees, had used Section 24 funds to employ specialist scheme staff, to contribute to the salaries of support staff in hostels managed by housing associations and, in one instance, to secure quotas of hostel places.

However, while a range of accommodation options is required, this should not be at the expense of policies that recognise the importance of a flexible, needs-led approach to leaving care. The expectation that young people should move on at such an early age is unrealistic and the minority who were able to remain with carers until they felt ready to leave 'home' were, perhaps, the most privileged of all. Only a handful of young people in our study were able to remain in placements beyond the age of 18 if needed, and this happened only where creative use of funding under Section 24 of the Children Act was used to convert foster placements to supported lodgings. A recent inspection has found that, despite many young people wanting fostering or very supported lodgings before moving to more independent accommodation, these resources appear to be in short supply (Social Services Inspectorate 1997).

Flexibility should also involve an opportunity for young people to return to more supported accommodation when necessary. It is not uncommon for young people who have left their family home to return home and later leave again, so that in effect they leave home more than once (Banks *et al.* 1992; Jones 1995). This process involves shifts from dependence to independence and back again. For care leavers, however, the provision of respite is rare. In our study, it appeared to be an option available only to some young people with learning difficulties or to young mothers where there were concerns about the child. However, a number of other young people experienced crises that placed them at risk of further instability, including homelessness, and would have benefited from a return to a more supported option. An approach which allows for care leavers to return to more sheltered accommodation when needed could contribute to a more successful transition in the long term.

Finally, the provision of accommodation is unlikely to be sufficient without an offer of ongoing support until young people no longer need it or develop an alternative network of support. Although many of the care leavers in our study were in contact with their parents, very few had positive relationships with them or received a great deal of support from them, so they were obliged to rely on professional support. Many young people lacked the skills and confidence to manage their homes without support and others encountered crises at a later point. The 'housing plus support' approach of leaving care schemes was also a major factor in increasing tenancy allocations. Housing providers were more likely to take a risk on a young person if support plans were in place and negotiated with them. A vital element of successful transitions, therefore, is the provision of ongoing support commensurate with the needs of individual young people for as long as they require it.

CONCLUSION

Leaving care, although a pivotal moment in the lives of looked-after young people, needs to be understood in the context of the broader transitions to adulthood undertaken by young people in the 1990s. As we have seen, traditional pathways to adulthood have been profoundly restructured in recent years and this process has been reinforced by social policies which both assume and reinforce a pattern of young people remaining longer within the family home. Early exposure to the uncertainties of the labour and housing markets can carry greater risks for young people, especially for those compelled to leave home at 16 or 17 and who lack continuing family support. In this context, care leavers – a group made vulnerable by their past experiences – are particularly disadvantaged. The majority are expected to move to independence at this age, most fail to obtain qualifications, experience genuine difficulties finding employment and, in consequence, are often required to cope with the pressures of multiple transition whilst subsisting at or below benefit levels. Their over-representation amongst samples of the young homeless is therefore not surprising.

The Children Act does offer a framework for providing a comprehensive range of services to young people leaving care and, at least potentially, for responding to the not dissimilar needs of homeless teenagers. However, as we have seen, it does suffer from two areas of weakness. First, the balance of duties and powers within it, especially in relation to financial assistance, has meant that the uneven development of leaving care services has continued. The kind of service a young person receives still tends to depend on where they happen to live. None the less the Act has served to raise the profile of leaving care and sponsored the development of a range of more specialist services. Second, its implementation has coincided with a raft of social policies that have had an adverse effect on the transition possibilities of young people and which social care workers have been able to do little about.

Services for care leavers and for other vulnerable young people who leave home at an early age therefore need to form part of a broader integrated set of youth policies designed to support young people's transitions to adulthood. At a minimum, these policies should recognise that certain categories of young people have little choice but to leave home early and that, for these groups, negotiating later family support is likely to prove difficult. At national and local levels the development of inter-departmental strategies is required to promote appropriate accommodation options, adequate incomes, access to employment and training opportunities and social support. Without such a package, of which the provisions of the Children Act form just one part, the risks and uncertainties to which these young people are exposed are unlikely to diminish.

Chapter 7

Youth homelessness

Nicholas Pleace and Deborah Quilgars

This chapter is concerned with youth homelessness and draws particularly on the last major survey of single homelessness conducted
in England (Anderson *et al.* 1993). The first section of the chapter
examines the different causes of youth homelessness. The following
section considers the issues around defining and measuring youth
homelessness in Britain. The final section examines the experiences
and characteristics of young homeless people in Britain during the
1990s. The conclusion examines some of the issues surrounding
effective intervention to counteract and prevent youth homelessness,
a theme that is considered in more detail in the next chapter.

THE CAUSES OF YOUTH HOMELESSNESS

In common with the more general literature on the causes of homelessness (Neale 1997; Pleace 1998b) studies of youth homelessness
have drawn attention to the role of individual characteristics. The
first serious research into homelessness questioned the traditional
stereotype of the homeless person as an individual who had actively
chosen their situation, and instead emphasised individual vulnerability – usually poor health status – as the cause (NAB 1966;
Greve 1971). Since the late 1980s, work on homelessness has stressed
that many of those who experience it are vulnerable in ways that
predispose them to being especially open to structural factors that
precipitate homelessness, such as changes in housing supply or
labour markets (Dant and Deacon 1989). When work specifically
concerned with youth homelessness appeared, it focused on the
inability of some young people to cope with managing life on their
own because they were both vulnerable and unprepared.

Youth homelessness among people aged 16–24 is strongly associated with past experience of child protection and childcare services, as discussed in detail by Biehal and Wade (this volume). Hutson and Liddiard (1994) and Ploeg and Scholte (1997) have also noted that a disrupted childhood with experiences of fostering or care make it much more likely that a young person will enter homelessness. Less than 1 per cent of young people enter care in the UK and yet the proportions of young people with experience of care are between 25 per cent and 30 per cent whenever homeless people are surveyed (Hutson and Liddiard 1994: 60). However, youth homelessness cannot be explained simply in terms of the experience of care leavers. Some young people leave home because of family conflict (particularly if a parent has changed partners), because a parent or parents are no longer willing to support them, or because they are escaping violence or abuse (Jones 1995b). These young people are not necessarily any better equipped than those leaving care to cope with independent living and may enter homelessness for that reason. However, while the inability of some young people to manage to live independently is clearly a key factor in causing youth homelessness, it is also important to consider the causal impact of political decisions and changes in society.

In 1979, the first of a succession of Conservative governments was elected which had a right-wing ideology grounded in nineteenth-century ideas about the role of the state and the individual. These governments emphasised 'traditional' family structures (regardless of the fact that they had actually become much less common), individual responsibility and a free market ethos. Successive benefit cuts that reduced the eligibility of under-25s for assistance placed a greater stress on family support for young adults, reducing their ability to compete in the housing market (Jones and Wallace 1992; Rugg, this volume). In addition, as the consequence of a series of housing policy initiatives, the Conservative governments instituted a massive reduction in the supply of affordable social housing for rent. This decrease occurred through the introduction of the Right to Buy which allowed tenants to purchase the houses they had been renting from councils, and through the effective end of the government subsidy that had allowed councils to build new stock. Emphasis was instead placed on reduced funding to the much smaller housing association sector. With the introduction of private finance into the development of new build by housing associations in the 1988 Housing Act, even this small sector lost much of its capacity to build properties that were affordable to people on low incomes (Pleace *et al.* 1998). Furthermore, it was unclear how far attempts to revive the declining private rented sector were meeting with success (Crook *et al.* 1995). As a consequence of both housing and welfare policies, therefore, young people without secure well-paid employment were faced with both an absolute shortage of housing to rent and an inability to afford what may be on offer (Anderson 1994; Prescott-Clarke *et al.* 1994; Hutson and Liddiard 1994).

Carlen (1996) has taken the view that the attitude of the Conservative governments of the 1980s and 1990s to young home-less people was so hostile that it could be interpreted as one of the central causes of youth homelessness. She argues that the refusal of the state to assist young people who were homeless was con-ditioned by a simplistic ideological response to complex social problems, which was essentially to blame the group experiencing problems for their own circumstances. In this view, the end of signi-ficant support for the social rented sector and changes to the social security system helped cause increased youth homelessness and yet the government of the day reacted to it by attacking the young people who experienced homelessness: 'The most effectively accom-modating narrative recasts the young unemployed and homeless as being socially expendable, but presently threatening products of a corrosive "dependency culture" spawned by an always and already inept welfarism' (Carlen 1996: 42–3).

An alternative perspective is that what the Conservative govern-ments did was in some senses inevitable, as massive public expendi-ture by the developed world became unsustainable in the face of competition from the developing world (OECD 1996). From this perspective, the great loss of full-time employment and shift to hypercasualisation (more part-time work than ever before, dis-proportionately undertaken by women, combined with the loss of unskilled full-time jobs) over which the Conservatives presided in the 1980s and 1990s was unavoidable (Jordan 1996). The general downturn in full-time unskilled employment provided the final diffi-culty for young people who were in danger of becoming homeless, as it would become increasingly difficult for them to find well-paid work. The increasing evidence that some young people were being caught in a Catch-22 situation of 'no home, no job', and more general evidence of increasing youth unemployment, was one of the main reasons for the development of the Foyer movement, designed to address youth homelessness and unemployment, under the Conservatives (Anderson and Quilgars 1995; Quilgars and Pleace, this volume). Under the current Labour government, a specific focus on youth unemployment is part of the welfare to work programmes referred to as the 'New Deal', and the focus of the Social Exclusion Unit on youth homelessness shows that concern with the problem continues.

In reality, as Neale (1997) has demonstrated, there is no single cause of homelessness and it is a misunderstanding of the nature of this social problem to attempt to look for some sort of universal truth about it, other than perhaps seeing it as the extreme result of the more general processes causing social and economic marginal-isation in society (Pleace 1998b). Clearly, individual experience plays an important role because of what is known about the relation-ship between severe disruption to family life leading to intervention by social services and the rates of homelessness among young people with such a background. The low economic status of the households into which young people who become homeless are generally born is also important in influencing their life chances (Ploeg and Scholte 1997). At the same time, Carlen's view of youth homelessness as being increased because of the ideology of successive Conservative governments, while perhaps exaggerated, points to policy changes that almost certainly increased youth homelessness. Those research-ers who emphasise the role of housing supply, such as Anderson (1994), also make an important contribution to the discussion of youth homelessness. The actual cause of each young person's homelessness is the result of complex interaction between context, characteristics, experience and, quite possibly, an element of chance.

The following section is concerned with defining youth homeless-ness and measuring the scale of the problem. The remainder of the chapter considers the needs and characteristics of young people who experienced homelessness in Britain during the 1990s.

DEFINING AND MEASURING YOUTH HOMELESSNESS

Youth homelessness is a widespread and visible problem in some cities and many services have been developed to counteract it. Thousands of young people are in projects for homeless people (Pleace et al. 1998) and in 1995, according to the then Department of the Environment quarterly statistics, local authorities rehoused

3,500 vulnerable young people under the terms of the homelessness legislation. Estimates produced by the voluntary sector range from 33,000 homeless 16–21 year olds in the UK (London Research Centre 1996) to 246,000 homeless 16–25 year olds (Evans 1996), although these figures are not the result of systematic research and are, in essence, little more than guesses. Almost all young people leave home either to get married or live with a partner or to undertake a degree or some other educational qualification (Jones 1995b), but it is certain that each year at least several thousand join the homeless population.

However, while it is possible to be able to state without hesitation that the UK has a significant social problem in the form of youth homelessness, precisely describing and measuring that problem is very difficult. The main difficulty arises from the way in which the homelessness legislation works in the UK. In broad terms (Anderson, this volume) the division is based on perceived ability to function in society without assistance: thus homeless children and people who are 'vulnerable' under the terms of the law therefore receive assistance from the state. Those who are deemed capable of securing accommodation are essentially left to fend for themselves, although local authorities have a duty to provide advice and assistance.

Young homeless people are divided by the legislation into those who are statutorily homeless and those who are non-statutorily homeless (generally referred to as single homeless people). The boundaries between these populations are vague, as someone accepted as statutorily homeless in one locality may be refused assistance in another (Anderson and Morgan 1997). The extent of the non-statutorily homeless population of young people is also open to dispute because of disagreements about exact definitions of 'homelessness'. Some commentators argue that almost any form of housing need can be referred to as homelessness, and may define a teenager's wish to live independently from their parents as 'hidden homelessness'. Such definitions are ultimately unhelpful, since they do not differentiate between a wish to move from perfectly adequate housing, severe housing need, and the situation of homeless people who literally have nowhere suitable to live. Government and homelessness professionals tend to take the view that anyone living on the streets or in an institution for homeless people or in other *temporary* accommodation is homeless (for example, official statistics generally treat young people and others living in bed and breakfast hotels or hostels as homeless). This definition does not include anyone who is living in private rented or housing association housing on a time limited contract, as they are regarded as securely housed. Popular and media views of homelessness tend to be restricted only to those people who are sleeping rough.

Academics, the voluntary sector and government have yet to agree on a definition of youth homelessness or homelessness in general in the UK. This situation creates a context in which any attempted measurement of the problem is instantly a political statement, in the sense that the definition employed for the measurement is likely to conflict with the working definitions of youth homelessness used by at least some other agencies. To this difficulty is added the practical problems of trying to count a population that is dynamic, because people enter and leave youth homelessness, temporarily and permanently, every day (Anderson *et al.* 1993; Hutson and Liddiard 1994). Young homeless people may also be difficult to find if they are living on the streets or in squats or in any setting that does not keep accurate records. There is also some evidence to suggest that some young homeless people are highly mobile (Pleace 1998a).

THE CHARACTERISTICS OF YOUNG HOMELESS PEOPLE IN ENGLAND

In 1990, the Department of the Environment (now the Department of Environment, Transport and the Regions) commissioned the Centre for Housing Policy (CHP) at the University of York to undertake a large-scale survey of single homeless people in England. At that time, concern about street homelessness was increasing and, in particular, attention was becoming focused on the number of young people experiencing homelessness. At the time of writing, the 1991 Survey conducted by CHP remains the only large-scale rigorous survey of single homelessness carried out since 1981 in England. The survey included a large sample of single homeless people living in hostels and bed and breakfast hotels (B&Bs) and two smaller samples of people sleeping rough.

At that time, the proportion of young people among the rough sleeping or street homeless population was increasing, but the great majority of people sleeping rough were white, middle aged and male (Anderson *et al.* 1993). Although there is limited evidence of a further increase in the representation of young people, and particularly young women, among people sleeping rough, the population is still largely white, middle aged and male (Pleace 1998a). The majority of data on young people from the 1991 survey therefore came from that element of the survey that examined people living in B&Bs and hostels: a total of 392 young people were found in this group.

Table 7.1 shows the breakdown of the hostel and B&B sample from the survey by age. Compared with the population of adults in Britain at that time, people aged under 25 were over-represented amongst single homeless people in hostels and B&Bs. The most recent census at the time the data were collected showed that 18 per cent of the general population were 16–24 year olds, compared with 30 per cent of the single homeless people living in hostels. In contrast, the smaller numbers of young people found among the two samples of people sleeping rough were closer to the proportion of 16–24 year olds found in the general population (15 per cent and 19 per cent respectively).

Women are generally less likely to be part of the single homeless and rough sleeping population than men. However, when the survey data were examined it was found that women were disproportionately found among younger people who were homeless. Nearly two-fifths (38 per cent) of people aged under 25 were women, compared to less than a fifth of single homeless people who were over 25 (17 per cent).

Young people who were homeless were also a great deal more likely than the general population to be from an ethnic minority background. These findings were to some extent influenced by the urban and particularly the London focus of the 1991 survey,

Table 7.1 Single homeless people in hostels and B&Bs by age

Age	Number	Percentage
16–17	65	5
18–24	324	26
25–44	464	37
45–59	232	18
60+	181	14
Total	1,266	100

Source: Anderson et al. (1993)

although this focus was itself the product of single homelessness being concentrated in these areas. Forty per cent of single homeless people aged under 25 who were living in B&Bs and hostels were from ethnic minority backgrounds, compared to 20 per cent of those over 25 living in the same situation. At that time, people from ethnic minorities represented only 5 per cent of the general population (Office of National Statistics 1998).

In common with other single homeless people, the young people in B&Bs and hostels were almost all economically inactive. Only 12 per cent were in work the week preceding their interview, 49 per cent were looking for work and 16 per cent were not currently looking for work. A small per centage of young people were full-time students and 11 per cent of 16–17 year olds were on government training schemes. Reliance on benefits for income was correspond-ingly high, with 44 per cent of young people aged 16–17 and 60 per cent of those aged 18–24 having received Income Support in the last week and approximately two-thirds of young people receiving Housing Benefit. Begging was not usually mentioned as a source of income, except by some young people who were in the samples of people sleeping rough. Average income rose with age, with young people receiving a median income of £31 a week (figures are for 1991), rising to £40 a week for those aged 25–60 and £53 for people aged over 60 and this reflected the age-banded structure of Income Support. Qualitative material from focus groups that were also conducted as part of the 1991 survey indicated that some 16–17 year olds encountered such difficulties in trying to claim Income Support following the rule changes removing their entitlement in 1988 that they relied on begging and other sources of income instead.

Table 7.2 shows the experience that young people in hostels and B&Bs had of living in various institutional settings. As other research has also demonstrated, the 1991 survey showed that many homeless young people, particularly those aged 16–17, had stayed in a children's home or with foster parents at some stage in their lives. Among those aged 16–17, 39 per cent had stayed in a children's home and 32 per cent with foster parents. In contrast, 18 per cent of those aged 18–24 had stayed in a children's home and 11 per cent with foster parents. While significant numbers of older people living in hostels and B&Bs (12 per cent and 8 per cent respectively) had experience of children's homes or foster parents, the figures were lower than those for young people.

Table 7.2 Institutional settings experienced by hostel and B&B residents

Setting	16–24 (%)	25 and over (%)	All (%)
Children's home	22	12	15
Foster parents	15	8	10
General hospital*	3	13	10
Psychiatric hospital†	6	15	12
Alcohol unit	2	10	7
Drugs unit	4	2	3
Young offenders' unit	14	7	9
Prison or remand	20	27	25
Any institution	42	50	47

Source: Anderson et al. (1993).

Notes: * For more than three months, † or psychiatric unit; percentages are rounded

Table 7.2 also shows that a fifth of young people had been in prison or a remand centre and that 14 per cent had been in a young offenders' institution. As would be expected among single homeless people, there was a much higher rate of stays in psychiatric units or hospitals than would be found among the general population (Pleace and Quilgars 1996). Overall, 42 per cent of 16–24 year olds had stayed in one or more institutions, or been fostered – a very high figure bearing in mind their young age. The survey also included some questions on health and access to medical services. It was found that while the majority of young people living in hostels or B&Bs were registered with a doctor, the youngest group (people under 18) were much more likely (77 per cent) than those aged 18–24 to report a health problem (54 per cent).

A third of young people had been living in their hostel or B&B for less than a month and nine out of ten had lived there for less than a year. Older single homeless people were likely to have been in their accommodation for longer periods of time. Young people were most likely to have been staying with friends or relatives (32 per cent) before they moved into their B&B or hostel, although 11 per cent had been staying with their parents and 16 per cent had been in night shelters or another hostel. Another 16 per cent reported that they had been sleeping rough before entering the hostel and almost half (46 per cent) reported having slept rough in the last twelve months. Young people were more likely to have slept rough in the last year than people in the older age groups (46 per cent compared to 37 per cent), reflecting the tendency of the older people to have been in their accommodation for longer. Very few rough sleepers habitually sleep outside: both younger and older people tend to experience periods of rough sleeping in between stays in temporary accommodation and sometimes return to rough sleeping after periods in 'permanent' housing (Anderson *et al.* 1993; Vincent *et al.* 1995; Pleace 1995; Pleace 1998a). This pattern of rough sleeping reflects the haphazard access that people sleeping rough have to some direct access (first come, first served) hostels or shelters and other forms of accommodation and the inability of some to live independently without support after securing access to permanent housing.

Single homeless people aged over 24 were much more likely than young homeless people to have left their last settled home more than six months ago (42 per cent compared with 18 per cent). This tendency for young homeless people to have been homeless for shorter periods can also be seen in the finding that 62 per cent of this group had lived in their last settled home less than a year before they were surveyed, in comparison with only 33 per cent of people aged over 24. Nearly half of the young people (45 per cent) said that their last settled home had been their parents' home, although 15 per cent said that their last home had been with friends or relatives and 13 per cent considered their current B&B or hostel as being their home. People aged over 24 were obviously more likely to report that their last home had been their own (41 per cent), although 20 per cent said that their last home had been their parents'.

As other research has indicated, the survey found that quite a high proportion of young people had left home because of parental conflict (14 per cent), relationship breakdown (6 per cent), or abuse or violence (3 per cent). However, 8 per cent had left to look for work, 5 per cent because of eviction, and 5 per cent because of harassment or feeling insecure in their last home. Again, as other work has shown, no one reason or set of reasons for leaving their last settled home predominated.

The majority of young people appeared not to have given up hope of finding somewhere to live as 70 per cent of them said they were currently looking for accommodation, compared to 50 per cent of those aged over 24. Table 7.3 shows the actions that single homeless people living in hostels and B&Bs had taken to find accommodation, and it can be seen that young people were consistently more likely than those aged over 24 to be actively seeking accommodation.

Table 7.3 Action taken to find accommodation

Action	16–24 (%)	25 and over (%)
Approached council as homeless	45	33
On a council/housing association list	47	31
Approached advice agency	23	13
Looked for private rented housing	38	26
Asked friends/relatives if could stay	36	16
Done something else	16	10
At least one of the above	82	60

Source: Anderson et al. (1993)

Note: Refers to whether action(s) taken in the last 12 months

Almost all young people (95 per cent) would have preferred to live in a house or flat and only 1 per cent wanted to return to their parents. Although many had stayed with friends or relatives in the last year, none of the young people said that this arrangement was their preferred accommodation. Single homeless people over 24 were less likely than the younger group to want their own house or flat (79 per cent) and more likely to want to stay in the hostel or B&B they currently occupied (12 per cent). Most young people wanted their own place (either living alone or with their partner), rather than sharing accommodation (76 per cent). A high proportion of both young people (71 per cent) and people over 24 (79 per cent) expressed a preference to live alone. However, as Table 7.4 shows, young people were more likely than people over 24 to want some support if they were going to live alone.

Table 7.4 Need for support in preferred accommodation by age

Support	16–17 (%)	18–24 (%)	25–59 (%)	60+ (%)
Housekeeping/money management	62	30	23	33
Companionship	38	28	26	33
Medical help	17	13	17	34
Advice	55	40	34	38
Social work help	41	23	24	35
Other	3	6	8	4

Source: Anderson et al. (1993)

Six out of ten people aged under 18 and three out of ten people aged between 18 and 24 said that they would need help with housekeeping or money management. As is shown in Table 7.4, just over two-fifths of people under 18 (41 per cent) and almost a quarter of those aged between 18 and 25 (23 per cent) also said that they would need social work help. The youngest age group were the most likely to require support if they were going to live independently. Again, these findings echo those of other research into single homelessness which has emphasised that many single homeless people, both younger and older, require a range of support as well as housing if they are to manage living independently (Dant and Deacon 1989; Vincent et al. 1995; Pleace 1995).

No large-scale academic survey work on the characteristics of people sleeping rough and single homeless people in England has been completed since the survey conducted by Anderson et al. in 1991. However, the voluntary sector, which provides considerable assistance to single homeless people and people sleeping rough, continued to collect data throughout the 1990s. Figures collected by organisations like CRASH (1996) indicated that the increase in the number of young people, and in particular young women, among single homeless people and people sleeping rough continued through the decade.

In 1996/7 work was undertaken in conjunction with Crisis with funding from the Joseph Rowntree Foundation to evaluate a series of nightshelters called Open Houses that Crisis had established in five small cities and towns in England (Pleace 1998a). As part of this work, basic statistical information on the residents of these five schemes was collected and this provided details on 1,458 single homeless people and people sleeping rough. This piece of work was not a systematic survey of the single homeless and rough sleeping populations in the way that the work of Anderson et al. was, because it was confined simply to the residents of the five schemes rather than the population as a whole. However, the work did provide some basic details on 404 young people who used the five nightshelters.

The information from the five Open Houses indicated that there may have been some further increase in the proportion of young people and young women among single homeless people and people sleeping rough. Twenty-nine per cent of all residents were under 25 years old and 6 per cent were under 18. These figures were comparable with the hostel and B&B sample surveyed by

Anderson *et al.* However, since the Open Houses were used primarily by people sleeping rough it is perhaps more logical to compare it with the two smaller samples of people sleeping rough that Anderson *et al.* surveyed, which found that between 15 per cent and 19 per cent of people sleeping rough were under 25 years old.

As would be expected in a population with high levels of experience of rough sleeping (72 per cent of Open House residents had slept rough the night before or one or more times during the last year), women were relatively unusual and comprised only 12 per cent of residents. However, the same tendency as Anderson *et al.* found for women to be more strongly represented among the younger age groups was repeated in the data from 1996/7: 32 per cent of residents aged under 18 were women, compared with 20 per cent of residents aged 18–24 and just 9 per cent of residents aged 25–59.

The ethnic origin of the people staying in the Open Houses was similar to that of the two samples of people sleeping rough surveyed in Anderson *et al.* Less than 2 per cent of Open House residents were Black or Asian. There is strong evidence from Anderson *et al.* and official statistics that people from ethnic minorities are over-represented in the young single homeless populations who are not sleeping rough but who are living in hostels and other temporary accommodation in urban areas.

The data from the evaluation of Open House also reinforced the findings of Anderson *et al.* with regard to experience of rough sleeping. Young people were less likely to have experience of prolonged rough sleeping, but almost as likely to have spent at least some time sleeping rough as the other age groups. The Open House evaluation also found that young people were more likely than other age groups to have been homeless for very short periods. Sixty-seven per cent of people under 18 had only been homeless for a week or less and 55 per cent of people aged 18–24 fell into this same category. These percentages compared with just 30 per cent of people aged 25 and over. Again, these data also point to the erratic and sometimes temporary nature of rough sleeping by young homeless people, as is found among the population of people sleeping rough as a whole (Anderson *et al.* 1993).

Findings from the Open House data were also broadly comparable with those of Anderson *et al.* with regard to health status and access to health services, although the Open House data also indicated a difference between older and younger people in one respect.

Young people aged between 18 and 24 were more likely than other age groups to report a drug addiction (12 per cent compared to 4 per cent of people under 18 and 8 per cent of people aged 25 to 44). *None* of the residents over the age of 45 reported a drug addiction, but they were more likely than younger age groups to report dependency on alcohol.

The Open House evaluation also examined the mobility of homeless people, asking them how long they had lived in the area before arriving at an Open House. There was marked variation between the mobility of the different age groups. Young people were much less likely than other age groups to have just arrived in the town where an Open House was located. Under a fifth of people under 18 (18 per cent) had arrived in the area the same night as they first stayed in an Open House, compared to 34 per cent of people aged 18–24. In contrast, 41 per cent of people aged 25 to 44 and half the people aged 45 and over arrived in town on the same night that they first stayed in an Open House. Half the young people aged under 18 reported that they had always lived in the town where the Open House they were staying in was located, compared to 22 per cent of people aged 18–24 and 16 per cent of the other age groups.

The data collected for the Open House research do seem to confirm the findings of the comprehensive survey conducted by Anderson *et al.* in 1991 and also indicate that the characteristics and experience of young people who are homeless have not undergone significant change during the 1990s. As well as underlining the continued importance of the 1991 survey to our understanding of youth homelessness at the turn of the century, the data from the Open House evaluation (alongside other more recent research material referred to above) also demonstrate some evidence of prolonged policy failure, as young people continue to join the homeless population.

The research evidence suggests that there are important differences between young people who are homelessness and other groups in the homeless population. The most important of these differences – the association between experience of care and fostering and youth homelessness – is discussed in detail by Biehal and Wade in this volume. As would be expected, overall experience of homelessness is less than for other groups and there is some evidence that young people are less likely to travel away from the place in which they have grown up than other people in the rough sleeping population. However, the intermittent experience of rough sleeping among young people reflects the patterns found elsewhere in the homeless population. It would be wrong to characterise young people who are homeless as any more or less vulnerable or in need of assistance than any other group in the homeless population, although projects for young people tend to outnumber those for other groups in the single (or non-statutorily) homeless population (Pleace and Quilgars 1996). Nevertheless, all the indications are that this is a highly vulnerable group of young people who are often in urgent need of assistance.

CONCLUSION

There is some evidence that overall levels of rough sleeping are declining following the impact of the Rough Sleeper's Initiative, and the numbers of statutory acceptances under the terms of the homelessness legislation have also fallen. Despite these changes, the problem of homelessness and youth homelessness remains and there is at least anecdotal evidence from the voluntary sector and other organisations that youth homelessness may even be forming a relatively greater element within the homeless population.

Clearly, the context in which youth homelessness rose to the highest levels for some decades has recently been subject to changes which may become important in causing the overall level to decline. The emphasis on the social exclusion of youth and developments like the Social Exclusion Unit and the New Deal, alongside the Foyer initiative introduced under the Conservatives, could create a situation in which more services and more options are available to marginalised or vulnerable young people, which in turn may prevent entry into homelessness. At the same time, many of the central elements of public policy, such as the 1988 changes to Income Support and the recent single room rent changes in Housing Benefit, remain in place and increases in investment in social housing and associated services, while they are now occurring, will never mean a return to the levels of expenditure seen in the early 1970s. It does also have to be accepted that the extent to which a national government can control economic change or cushion its citizens from changes in the global economy is rather more limited than it once was, and the possibility of some young people facing low status employment and in a few instances permanent unemployment has to be recognised (Jordan 1996; OECD 1996).

Intervention to prevent youth homelessness or to help young people out of youth homelessness is quite possible. There is sufficient research and sufficient evidence from successful projects in the voluntary and local authority sectors to demonstrate that with the right housing, practical support, social support and guidance, alongside access to education, training or work (as appropriate) young homeless people can be brought out of homelessness and kept out of it (Pleace 1995; Ploeg and Scholte 1997). There is also a broad consensus about the type of services that are desirable, which usually involves the provision of life skill training and support in a hostel designed to help young people 'move on', or support designed to help young people manage in their own tenancy and with other aspects of their lives.

This intervention is expensive as suitable accommodation and support must be provided, and in a few cases this support will need to be available on an open ended and perhaps even permanent basis if someone is not going to make a return to homelessness. Ultimately, the question for Britain, as for other industrialised nations, is whether the saving made from not devoting sufficient resources to the problem of youth homelessness is worth the social and moral cost, and loss of the potential, that results from individuals who are little more than children sleeping in shelters, hostels and on the street. The next chapter considers in detail the questions around policies and services designed to counteract and prevent youth homelessness.

Chapter 8

Housing and support services for young people

Deborah Quilgars and Nicholas Pleace

The previous chapter examined the nature of homelessness and its increase amongst young people. This chapter charts the development of services to meet the needs of these homeless young people and other young people in housing need. As will be seen, there has been a significant growth in housing and support services directed to this group of people, largely provided by the voluntary housing sector. The chapter begins by exploring the background to the expansion in services, before moving on to describe the spectrum of services which have been developed, particularly focusing on the role of transitional accommodation and resettlement services. Finally, the chapter reflects on the extent to which these services represent a co-ordinated and coherent pattern of services.

THE EVOLUTION OF SERVICES FOR YOUNG PEOPLE IN HOUSING NEED

During the 1980s, concern about the number of young people who were in housing need or experiencing homelessness began to increase. The social rented sector was constricting as many of the better local authority properties were sold under the Right to Buy and various government initiatives had failed to revive the private rented sector as a provider of affordable accommodation. In urban areas the social and sometimes the physical fabric of some local authority estates began to break down and large elements of the stock became difficult or near-impossible to let. At the same time, the economy was changing with full-time unskilled work being replaced by part-time, insecure and low-paid service sector employment. Young people without a great deal of education or training were finding it more difficult to secure both work and reasonable, affordable rented accommodation. Greater numbers of families were experiencing relative poverty as a succession of Conservative governments introduced policies that contributed towards the formation of a more polarised society. Although the rate of polarisation had lessened by the mid-1990s, British society is more unequal than it has been for 40 years (Hills 1998).

Some academics argue that the increase in relative poverty for some sections of the population was associated with greater familial tension in a context in which families were in any case becoming unstable because of various social changes. These tensions were reflected in a greater number of young people leaving home early, more runaways and also in greater levels of youth homelessness (Ploeg and Scholte 1997; Jones 1995b). Part of the reaction of a series of Conservative governments was to restrict the benefits available to young people to encourage them to stay at home. In a context in which reasonable affordable housing was becoming scarce and unskilled work was more difficult to find, this was – according to Carlen (1996) – a policy that was bound to create youth homelessness and a greater number of young people in housing need.

Yet by the early 1990s, youth homelessness and the housing needs of young people were increasingly being seen as a component of a wider compound disadvantage experienced by young people from socially and economically deprived backgrounds. Young people in housing need were not a homogeneous group, but this population contained disproportionate numbers of young people who had been in care or who had had a disrupted childhood. In addition the young people in housing need or who were homeless, overwhelmingly came from socio-economically deprived sections of society (Ploeg and Scholte 1997; Hutson and Liddiard 1994; Pleace and Quilgars, this volume). Under the Conservatives in the 1990s and under the Labour government elected in 1997, excluded young people were increasingly seen as being one of the leading social problems faced by British society. Perhaps the single most important move to counteract this social problem under the Conservatives was their support for the Foyer programme, while Labour has introduced various schemes and programmes, the most significant being the New Deal. At the same time, throughout the 1990s and in the absence of statutory homelessness legislation which was able to meet the needs of single homeless young people, the voluntary sector became champions for addressing the cause of youth homelessness, increasingly being successful in raising finance for many initiatives, programmes and services designed to address youth homelessness and housing need.

By the mid-1990s something of a consensus or broad orthodoxy about how to help young people in housing need was emerging. Developing services were tending to concentrate on the following areas:

- *Housing need.* There was obviously a concern to meet the requirements of young people for affordable accommodation of a reasonable standard. Some schemes provided accommodation, at least on a temporary basis, while others helped young people secure access to semi-independent or independent tenancies. As well as providing shelter, such accommodation would also have to contain the basic necessities for living, such as some furniture and kitchen equipment, especially if young people were setting up home for the first time.
- *Daily living skills.* Young people may leave their parental home, foster care or a children's home quite unequipped for independent living. Some schemes aim to train young people how to cook, manage bills and generally run a home before they move into an independent or semi-independent tenancy; others aim to provide support following the initial move.
- *Employment and training.* As youth housing need and homelessness are seen as one manifestation of wider social and economic exclusion, the incorporation of young people into the formal economy is a priority of many projects.

In addition to focusing on these core areas, some schemes and services adopt a wider remit, particularly if they are designed for 'vulnerable' young people and also consider the following needs in their service provision:

- *Social care and health care needs.* Young people are less likely than the rest of the population to have serious health problems, but young people who are in housing need or who are homeless have often had negative life experiences. They may sometimes have mental health problems associated with their experiences prior to their housing need, such as experience of abuse (Jones 1995b; Ploeg and Scholte 1997). In addition, there is a high rate of dependency on drugs and alcohol among some groups of young homeless people (Gill *et al.* 1996), which may again be related to their experiences. If such needs are not addressed, young people may not be able to settle in a tenancy or secure work.

- *Social needs.* In some instances negative life experiences may make young people who are in housing need, or who are homeless, profoundly anti-social or withdrawn. Some services for young people in housing need concern themselves with social needs and may include elements of befriending or services designed to enhance social skills and the level of social interaction.
- *Financial needs.* Young people in housing need or who are homeless have restricted access to benefits and may find it difficult to secure work. Some schemes offer financial support by providing furniture or other necessities, may help organise benefit claims for their users, and/or help with finding deposits for rented accommodation.

This general consensus should not be seen as implying that there is a great deal of coherence in services for young people in housing need. While one project will be so comprehensive that the services it provides are basically open ended in terms of meeting the needs of the young people who use it, another will confine itself to a narrow definition of meeting the housing needs of young people. Other services are halfway between these relative extremes. As the rest of the chapter will show, not only do services provide different elements of support from one another but the nature of the voluntary sector developments at a local level has meant that projects with the same focus have often adopted different models of service delivery. While it is true that there was a broad consensus as to what the problem was and how to deal with it, when individual agencies began to work on projects for young people in housing need a diversity of projects and services began to appear.

PATTERNS OF SERVICE PROVISION

The broad consensus or orthodoxy around services for young people has emerged in the 1990s despite the fact that housing and support services for young people have largely developed in a responsive, *ad hoc* manner at a local level. Whilst some large, typically national voluntary organisations can be seen to have been influential in the development of services for young people in housing need over the last decade, like Centrepoint and the Foyer Federation for Youth, much provision has been developed by small voluntary sector organisations working on a small locality basis. Given the diffuse nature of the evolution of services, to some extent, it is difficult to explain how such a strong consensus and direction has emerged in services. Yet despite an absence of co-ordination (see below), agencies throughout Britain have tended to focus on the provision of a similar range of services for young people in housing need.

The overriding emphasis has been on the provision of different forms of transitional accommodation for young people. Transitional accommodation includes any provision which is accessed by young people on a temporary basis. Services are usually delivered to young people which are to differing extents concerned with helping residents to move towards, or achieve the 'transition' from relative dependence to independence. Accommodation includes a spectrum of provision, with a range of short, medium and longer stay hostels, supported lodgings, shared houses or group homes and, increasingly, foyers for young people which place a particular emphasis on training and employment skills.

Some forms of transitional accommodation help young people to access semi-independent or independent accommodation; that is, they help young people with the process of resettling in the community. It is also possible to discern a second type of service, resettlement services, which are solely concerned with delivering help and support to young people in the move to independent living. The most commonly known type of resettlement service, which has begun to emerge in the second half of the decade, is floating support which is delivered to young people on a time-limited basis when they move into independent accommodation. Young people may of course either move through transitional accommodation to independence or directly into permanent housing. Access schemes have also increasingly been developed in the last five years to provide financial support with the payment of rent in advance and deposits to enable young people to move into private rented sector accommodation (Rugg 1996).

Whilst broad categories of different types of provision can be discerned, it is important to note that these services are rarely mutually exclusive: often a project will deliver a number of different services, for example providing hostel places, resettlement workers and the financial support of an access scheme. Also, most accommodation services necessarily provide housing advice and information on housing options, financial benefits, etc., in addition to specialist advice and information services, which are sometimes delivered as part of a youth centre or drop-in/day centre service. Most accommodation services are aimed at young people in housing need, generally, although a substantial amount of provision has also been developed for particular groups of young people – for example, young people leaving care (see Biehal and Wade, this volume) or young offenders.

Below, the role of transitional accommodation and resettlement services in meeting the needs of young people is examined in more detail.

Transitional accommodation: the panacea

No national datasets exist on the full range of transitional accommodation provided for people in housing need generally, or young people specifically. It is therefore impossible to give precise figures on the scale and growth of this type of provision for young people, nor accurately compare transitional accommodation with other types of provision for young people over the 1990s. None the less, the research and partial datasets which do exist overwhelmingly point to the increasing importance of this type of service and perhaps even a disproportionately high provision of services focused on youth within the homelessness sector.

The best source of comprehensive and up-to-date information on hostel provision is the London Hostels Directory produced annually by the Resource Information Service (RIS 1998). The London Hostels Directory lists over 26,000 bedspaces, including a full range of specialist accommodation for people with drug and alcohol problems, mental health problems, etc. Whilst being obviously confined to London, the directory still provides a useful reflection of the range of hostels seen throughout Britain. The directory allows an examination of the pattern of provision for young people by usefully listing the target age groups of all provision. The 1998 Directory characterised non-specialist schemes for homeless people into six main categories:

1 *Direct access*: hostels offering emergency places which homeless people can access immediately, with vacancies usually on a daily or at least weekly basis.
2 *Low support*: hostels providing only limited support, often in large premises.
3 *Medium support*: hostels/shared houses where staff are available during the day, but usually not on a 24-hour basis; emphasis on providing practical support and preparing for independent living.
4 *Supportive*: hostels/shared houses with a high staff-resident ratio, usually on 24-hour basis, providing a range of emotional and practical support including counselling, education and independent living skills.
5 *Foyers*: schemes for young people in housing need but with relatively low support needs which offer accommodation linked with employment and training services.
6 *Housing schemes*: includes flats, bedsits or shared houses providing both good quality housing and sensitive housing management, either offering permanent accommodation or a high likelihood of rehousing.

An analysis of these beds and schemes by target age range of provision reveals some interesting patterns in provision for young people *per se* and *vis-à-vis* provision for older homeless people.

Table 8.1 shows that 34 per cent of the 15,444 non-specialist beds available to homeless people in London were targeted to young people (defined as usually under aged 26, although sometimes under 30).

At first glance, this level of provision is perhaps not particularly surprising given the fact that young people are over-represented amongst single homeless people (see Pleace and Quilgars, this volume); however, it is quite high considering that there is no age restriction attached to access to the majority of the other beds, some of which will therefore be occupied by young people. In addition, nearly half of the number of schemes/organisations providing accommodation for homeless people exclusively target their services at young people. Whilst these two figures obviously reveal that young persons' projects, on average, tend to be smaller than those for older people, overall it may suggest a disproportionately high provision of services for young people as compared to older homeless people.

Table 8.1 Hostels for homeless people in London by target age group

Type of scheme	Number of schemes						Number of beds					
	Young people		All ages		Total		Young people		All ages		Total	
	(N)	(%)	(N)	(%)	(N)	(%)	(N)	(%)	(N)	(%)	(N)	(%)
Direct access	16	31	36	69	52	100	321	10	2,795	90	3,116	100
Low support	14	56	11	44	25	100	2,024	63	1,169	37	3,193	100
Medium support	63	56	49	44	112	100	1,154	41	1,631	59	2,785	100
Supportive	18	51	17	49	35	100	357	46	423	54	780	100
Foyers	8	100	–	–	8	100	824	100	–	–	824	100
Housing schemes	6*	24	19*	76	25*	100	560	12	4,186	88	4,746	100
Total	125	49	132	51	257	100	5,240	34	10,204	66	15,444	100

Source: Data collected from Resource Information Service (1998)

* Equals number of organisations offering this type of accommodation, rather than number of schemes

A closer examination of the breakdown of the different types of accommodation reveals that young persons' provision is very much concentrated within the transitional supported accommodation model, rather than at the emergency or more permanent housing end of the spectrum. Over 50 per cent of all low, medium support and supportive schemes are provided to young people, representing 63 per cent of low support beds, 46 per cent of supportive and 41 per cent of medium support provision. In addition, of course, 100 per cent of the foyer beds are available for young people, as considered below. In contrast, only 10 per cent of emergency beds are provided solely for young people, and 12 per cent of the housing scheme provision is targeted at younger groups (representing 31 per cent and 24 per cent of schemes/organisations).

A recent study of the housing needs of young people carried out for the Rural Development Commission (Ford *et al.* 1997) provides some useful information on the pattern of service provision in rural areas. A postal survey of rural district authorities, major charities and County Voluntary Youth Services revealed that most of the services that did exist for young people in housing need were also primarily concerned with meeting the temporary accommodation needs of young people. The provision of small hostels, shared housing and foyers was most prominent; however, again there were very few schemes concerned with the more routine need of young people for appropriate, permanent, self-contained accommodation. Overall there was a severe lack of provision of all types of services for young people in housing need. The study found that young people faced particular difficulties in accessing suitable housing in the rented sector in rural areas, and this, combined with other factors, often meant that young people had to move into towns or cities to access services.

A number of factors account for the predominance of transitional accommodation for young people: first, there is no doubt that specialist provision for young people has followed the existing pattern of emphasis on the provision of hostel accommodation for homeless people generally; second, funding sources, although problematic, have tended to be geared to supporting this type of provision; and third, part of the consensus or orthodoxy around service provision for young people is an assumption that young people need to be supported in the 'transition' from childhood to adulthood, and therefore require a more structured supportive environment through which to develop the skills for independent living. Perhaps finally it is also generally assumed that young people are naturally more suited than older people to living communally, and with their peer group. These last two factors are particularly important in explaining the development of foyers for young people.

Foyers for young people

Foyers for young people are undoubtedly the most prominent development in service provision for young people in the 1990s. When the idea was introduced to Britain, from France, by Shelter in 1992, it was greeted by a mixed response within the voluntary housing movement. Whilst many housing organisations, along with the government, felt that it represented a very positive opportunity to tackle both homelessness and unemployment, some commentators felt that foyers would mark an unhealthy return to large, institutional style hostels with draconian rules and regulations (see Housing press and Gilchrist and Jeffs 1995). Whilst Shelter and allied key organisations wanted to develop a network of 200 foyers by the year 2000, most people felt that foyers represented little more than the 'flavour of the month' and, particularly given funding difficulties, would never really become established in Britain as they had in France in the 1950s. Whilst Shelter's target of 200 is still a little way off, it is likely that there will be over a hundred foyers in operation by the Millennium. By the summer of 1998, 70 foyers were operational in the UK, with 34 in development, 56 planned and 103 speculative (Foyer Federation for Youth 1998a).

A pilot programme of foyers was set up in 1992 of five converted YMCA hostels (St Helens, Nottingham, Norwich, Wimbledon and Romford) and two new-build foyers developed by London and Quadrant Housing Trust and North British Housing Association (in Camberwell and Salford respectively) supported by both the Housing Corporation and the Employment Service. However, before the pilot programme was fully evaluated other foyers began to be developed, with the support of the newly formed Foyer Federation for Youth. Whilst the pilot foyers and many of the other foyers developed in the first few years of the initiative adopted the 'one large building' approach, by offering young people hostel-type accommodation and jobsearch/training resource facilities on site, foyers soon began to be developed to a variety of models to suit local needs and enable agencies to utilise existing resources. By 1996, over a third of foyers were in rural areas (Quilgars and

Anderson 1997), which gave an added impetus to the drive to develop smaller, innovative types of foyers. A number of foyers have been developed to a dispersed model, using a variety of different types of accommodation. For example, the Scarborough Home and Dry foyer combines training facilities and drop-in centre with private sector flats for young people with high support needs. The Richmond foyer also has a single training site with young people living in a number of shared houses. A recent initiative by Solon Wandsworth HA and Grenfell HA is using shortlife housing and linking up with Training and Enterprise Councils (TECs) and the Careers Service to provide training and employment opportunities.

It is difficult to measure the success of foyers. The pilot evaluation (Anderson and Quilgars 1995) found that foyers had successfully assisted many disadvantaged young people into training, employment and housing, but not necessarily in a linear way (i.e. young person undertaking training, securing a job and moving on to a permanent tenancy), and jobs were often low paid and/or of a temporary nature. Overall, foyers appear to provide a supportive environment where otherwise alienated young people can gain confidence to begin to make the transition towards independence. However, revenue funding remains a problem, often leading to affordability issues; securing move-on accommodation is still often difficult; and recent void problems in a number of foyers warn of the need to carry out detailed local needs surveys before setting up a foyer (Anderson and Douglas 1998; Foyer Federation for Youth 1998b). The Department of Environment, Transport and Regions has recently commissioned an evaluation of the outcomes of foyers which should provide more robust figures on the overall impact of the initiative. However, it cannot be denied that foyers have raised the profile of young people's services and the importance of adopting an integrated, holistic approach to meeting youth homelessness and unemployment.

It should also be noted that training and employment services are provided to homeless young people in a range of other settings as well as foyers. A recent publication (Community Partners 1998) identified 73 projects involved in training and employment for homeless people, many of which were targeted at young people, including training attached to hostels (for example, Centrepoint Vauxhall project), day centres like the London Connection, employment or job creation schemes such as the Big Issue and training agency based services (for example, Streets Ahead).

Resettlement services: a developing emphasis

While services for young homeless people are predominantly based in transitional accommodation, there have been some developments in resettlement services for young homeless people. Resettlement services first emerged when some large hostels for homeless single men were due for closure, and were initially designed to provide practical support and training for former residents who were presumed to be institutionalised and who would now be living independently (Dant and Deacon 1989). Quite soon afterwards local authorities and some housing associations that were experiencing high rates of abandonment and housing management problems when they let units to vulnerable single homeless people started to introduce resettlement services to reduce void levels. In most instances the remit was broadened and there was a focus on orchestrating the delivery of health and social services to formerly homeless people, as well as on some elements of practical and social support (Pleace 1995).

By the middle of the 1990s, some large urban local authorities with high levels of acceptances of young homeless people under the homelessness legislation were running resettlement services specifically for young people. As with resettlement services in general, these services developed in response to high levels of abandonment and other housing management problems. Sometimes these services were designed to function as part of a process which began with a stay in local authority transitional accommodation (also specifically targeted on young people) and ended with a move into an independent tenancy with a few months' support from a housing support or youth support worker. In other cases, young people would be moved straight into an independent tenancy but with a resettlement service visiting them for the first few months (Pleace 1995). Similar services began to be developed by the voluntary sector at about the same time as the Children Act came into effect, and local authority social services departments had new obligations towards young people leaving their care (Biehal and Wade, this volume).

Some local authority resettlement services for young homeless people are constrained by financial arrangements that require housing departments to spend their resources on housing services. Resettlement services for young homeless people operated by housing authorities cannot provide care because of these arrangements, and so only provide various forms of intensive housing management, including support in daily living skills and arranging access to other services, plus limited social support to help young people maintain their tenancy. More generally, the financial constraints under which housing authorities operate mean that funds are also highly limited, thus strictly rationing the time spent with each young person, both in terms of the hours of service each young person can receive and in the number of months that they are eligible for these services (Pleace 1995).

Resettlement services provided by the voluntary sector may be similarly constrained if they are wholly or partly funded by Housing Benefit. In this instance, rent officers have to determine whether the resettlement service in question is a legitimate use of the 'service charge' element of Housing Benefit before the service can be funded. However, once funding has been secured from Housing Benefit, or if it is secured from other sources (such as contracts from social services departments), the funding arrangements allow resettlement services provided by the voluntary sector to sometimes be more comprehensive than those provided by social landlords.

An example of such a service is the recently developed Capital Youth Link service, which has a wide remit concerned with all aspects of the welfare of the young people in housing need who use it. Unlike the resettlement services provided by social landlords, Capital Youth Link has an explicit objective to provide practical and *emotional* support to its 16- and 17-year-old users as they move into independent accommodation in Hackney. In common with other resettlement services for young people in housing need developed by voluntary sector organisations, the service is closer to that found in some transitional accommodation than to an intensive housing management service. Support in this instance is almost open ended, as workers will provide almost any assistance that the young people using the service require. The service, designed for vulnerable young people in housing need or who are homeless (England, forthcoming), is part funded by social services, but also supported by the Housing Corporation through Supported Housing Management Grant which represents another important funding source for this type of work.

Within the voluntary sector, which is largely funded in its activities through local authority and central government grants and contracts, a financial imperative is present in the development of resettlement services for young people in housing need and young homeless people. Transitional accommodation, whether it is a hostel, foyer or move-on accommodation, is relatively expensive. In contrast, a resettlement service based on travelling workers who support a number of young people in existing social rented or private rented flats can be operated relatively cheaply. The effectiveness of such services in comparison with transitional accommodation is difficult to determine because clear information on long-term effectiveness is thin on the ground. One study has suggested that such services can help prevent young homeless people abandoning a local authority tenancy in some instances (Pleace 1995).

CO-ORDINATING SERVICES: FROM SLOW BEGINNINGS...

When the demand for services to meet the housing needs of young people was growing in the late 1980s and early 1990s, the statutory services were neither given the resources nor the responsibility to respond to the problem. Consequently, the main impetus for service development was left to the voluntary housing movement. In many areas, the voluntary sector successfully championed the cause of meeting the needs of increasing numbers of young people in housing and social need, impressively patchworking services together and drawing on diverse and often problematic funding sources. However, at the same time, this response was often chaotic and unplanned. Service development was largely reliant on the existence of voluntary sector activity in an area and staff tenacity in identifying funding sources, rather than based on the identified need in an area. The effect of this has meant that some areas have better developed services than others, with some having no services at all. Services have tended to be developed more easily in urban settings and a resultant urban bias has led to problems of migration of young people from rural areas into towns and cities (Ford et al. 1997). There is also some evidence of incorrectly targeted provision due to an absence of locality planning of services.

Voluntary sector organisations have traditionally had little reason to communicate with each other and co-ordinate their activities. Having to compete for funding with each other has acted as a disincentive to working together. However, the planning of housing services for young people at a local level has been improving, if slowly at first, over the course of the 1990s. Local authorities, who have a duty to plan and oversee housing services, have taken an increasing interest in the needs of more vulnerable members of their community, in part spurred on by community care reforms and many policy directives on inter-agency working, although the extent of the involvement of voluntary sector providers and housing associations remains patchy. Many funding sources are now dependent on local authority support (for instance, Housing Corporation funding and the Single Regeneration Budget). Experience has shown the negative effects of ignoring needs assessment and planning, and many agencies are more cautious about developing potentially expensive services like foyers, commissioning feasibility studies to investigate local needs.

In addition, two major initiatives have been launched by national homelessness organisations to promote the development of regional or county strategies for tackling youth homelessness. In 1991, Centrepoint, with then Section 73 funding from the Department of the Environment, undertook a three-year pilot project to improve the housing options of young people in Oxfordshire. Two housing workers were employed to work with local agencies in mapping existing provision, identifying gaps, devising a strategy and putting this strategy into practice. The project contributed to the raising of £1.8 million for young people's projects in the county (Spafford 1994). The successful model was then replicated in Warwickshire and Devon, attracting funding from a range of governmental, charitable and commercial organisations. More recently, Shelter has adopted a very similar model known as the 'Network', with financial support from the Midland Bank, to employ workers in different areas to facilitate a co-ordinated approach to providing accommodation, advice and support services for young people, and ultimately to develop a methodology by which other areas can develop similar strategies. Following two years' research, the first Shelter Network reports were published in 1998 covering Lincolnshire (Stone 1998), Crawley/Horsham (Prime 1998) and South Yorkshire (Morton 1998).

The development of regional approaches to youth homelessness represents an important impetus to the better co-ordination of services for young people in housing need. However, in part, it unfortunately also illustrates the lack of communication and co-ordination which still exists, to an extent, at a national level. Whilst some initiatives, most prominently the recent Inquiry into Youth Homelessness (Evans 1996), have successfully involved many national agencies campaigning together on this issue, too often national voluntary agencies are still working independently of each other, competing for the same funding sources, in pursuit of very similar goals. However, the recent establishment of the Youth Homelessness Action Partnership (YHAP) by the Labour government, where major national youth homelessness charities along with key players in national and local government will meet and be involved in commissioning DETR research, could potentially represent a very significant development in co-ordinating activity in both the voluntary and statutory sector.

COHERENCE IN SERVICE PROVISION: DEFINITIONS AND STANDARDS

The lack of co-ordination in services for young people in housing need is largely an unintended result of the competitive environment in which the voluntary sector has had to develop services over the last decade. However, despite the existence of a consensus or ortho-doxy in service provision, the lack of co-ordination has inevitably led to something of a lack of coherence in the services for young people in housing need. Whilst services offer basically the same broad range of services, concerning themselves with social needs, support needs, training and educational needs, life skills and finan-cial needs, the detailed content and delivery of services can be quite different. For example, resettlement services for young people operate for different periods from between 6 weeks to 18 months, some emphasise practical support, others social support, some are concerned more with tenancy support than with the general quality of life of young people. Some services (e.g. Capital Youth Link) emphasise training and education within a broad remit, others are more focused on particular issues. In short, there is little acknowledgement within the sector of a need for service standards. Some services may be more consistently effective than others, but because so little robust research has been carried out on the long-term effectiveness of such provision it is impossible to know whether one model represents a more effective service for young people than another.

Transitional accommodation suffers from the same problems. For example, some schemes provide little more than enhanced housing management support, yet others offer intensive training and support for independent living. The emphasis on training, education and economic participation predominant in foyers is not always found in the other schemes. Other schemes may place a greater emphasis on life skills or other elements of preparation for independent living. Diversity within provision may ultimately be seen as a laudable aspect of housing provision for young people, but given the lack of information on effectiveness and coherence, the development of an overall strategy based on existing provision remains problematic.

Only very recently have some initiatives begun to be developed within the voluntary sector to address some issues of non-standardisation of services. For example, the Network to Advance Skills for Homeless People (NASHP), set up in 1998 by CRISIS, and the National Resettlement Agency set up by the National Homeless Alliance may both prove useful forums for the promotion of good practice and standards in such services. A National Rent Deposit Forum is also now in existence. In addition, the Foyer Federation for Youth is currently piloting an Accredited Foyer Status system which is attempting to reward high standards of service. There is clearly a drive towards voluntary sector self-regulation and promotion of good practice; however, there is still a long way to go before a coherent framework of services can be developed which can be supported with reference to proven standards in service delivery.

CONCLUSION

There is something of a policy disarray around responses to young people's housing need, but this cannot be blamed on the responses of the voluntary sector organisations who were placed in a situation in which they were competing with each other for various uncoordinated pots of government money. The rise of youth homelessness coincided with the general fragmentation of the welfare state as internal markets and quasi-markets were introduced by a succession of Conservative governments. However, the possibility that there is some imbalance in favour of transitional accommodation within the range of services for young people with housing needs in urban areas, alongside the general problem of a lack of co-ordination as well as a lack of information on activity, has made planning difficult, if not impractical. This situation has been exacerbated by the lack of coherence in service delivery by a range of disparate agencies, so it is uncertain who is providing which services, and the nature of the services being provided.

The moves by the voluntary sector to improve planning and co-ordination, although they need to be considered in a context of continued competition between such agencies rather than viewed as purely altruistic, may help this situation. The new emphasis on co-ordinated responses to social problems that has been a feature of New Labour may also help address this problematic situation.

Chapter 9

Housing and young single parent families

Suzanne Speak

This book is primarily concerned with the housing situation of young single people. However, in Britain, as in other European countries, there is an increasing number of young people who, although neither married nor cohabiting, are not thought of as single and often do not fit the criteria for single person's housing: they are the country's single young parents. Secondary analysis of the *Survey of English Housing* shows that 7 per cent of young women between the ages of 16 and 25 are single young mothers, with custody of and sole responsibility for their children. The number of single young fathers is tiny – much smaller than 1 per cent of men in that age group. The average age of single mothers in Britain is 25 years, but the group includes younger teenage mothers: around 4 per cent of young women aged 16–19 are lone parents. The increasing likelihood that young mothers will raise their children alone, rather than marrying or cohabiting with the father, leads to concern about single motherhood's cost to the state in terms of social housing and benefits. The 1990s saw a number of memorable political comments about young single mothers; for example, John Redwood commented in 1995: 'the assumption is that the illegitimate child is a passport to a council flat' (*Guardian* 14.8.95). After a number of studies of young single parenthood, there still remains no evidence that young people do consider a child in this way (Burghes and Brown 1995; Clark 1989; Speak *et al.* 1995, 1997).

Nevertheless, it is fair to say that two assumptions persist in the mythology surrounding young single parenthood. First, that the social housing system favours single parents over other families with children; and second, that affordable independent accommodation is the greatest need of single parents and the answer to

most of their problems. A number of research projects have dis-
proved these myths, and highlighted other issues which affect
single parents' lives, independence, housing, and ability to care for
their children. Many of the issues affecting the housing situation
of young people are structurally the same for parents and non-
parents. It is the impact of those issues, and a young person's ability
to adapt or overcome housing difficulties, which differs if a young
person has a dependent child. This chapter will consider those
differences.

Studies of young parenthood have primarily concentrated on
single young mothers. However, we should not disregard the fathers,
many of whom – although technically not custodial – do share some
level of responsibility for their children's upbringing, and who
society and politicians would have taking on greater responsibility.
Research is beginning to highlight the importance of housing in
maintaining relationships between children and their fathers after
divorce or separation, and there is no reason to assume the same
is not true for single, never-married fathers (Simpson *et al.* 1995;
Speak *et al.* 1997).

This chapter looks at the housing needs and aspirations of such
young parents and their children. It is not the intention to look
deeply into temporary accommodation, such as mother and baby
hostels, other than as a starting point on the route to longer-term
housing in its broader sense. Here we will consider the ways in
which young single parents differ from other young single people
without children, and how those differences govern their housing
situation. The chapter draws heavily on two recent qualitative
studies *Young Single Mothers: Barriers to Independent Living* (the
Independent Living Study – Speak *et al.* [1995]) and *Young Single
Fathers: their Participation in Fatherhood* (the Fatherhood Study –
Speak *et al.* [1997]). Both studies looked at the relationship between
disadvantage, housing and young single parents' abilities to establish themselves as independent adults caring for children. For the
Independent Living Study, 40 young single mothers were asked to
recount the difficulties they encountered in establishing and maintaining their first independent home. For the Fatherhood Study,
40 young single fathers were asked to discuss the barriers they
experienced to being involved in the care of their children. This
chapter is illustrated with the voices of the young parents interviewed for those studies.

BECOMING INDEPENDENT

The controversy surrounding young single mothers and their need for social housing wrongly assumes that their desire or need to establish their independence is specifically related to their status as parents. This is not so. Leaving home and becoming independent of one's family is a normal activity associated with growing up. Indeed, many of the mothers and fathers interviewed for the Independent Living Study and the Fatherhood Study were already living independently, or had applied for independent housing and were on local authority housing registers prior to becoming parents. The sudden and unplanned change of status of these young people simply made independence more urgent, and the maintenance and security of that independence more important. For those still living in the parental home there were, in some cases, difficult and unhappy relationships within the family, and the young people reported 'keeping out of the way' for much of the time. Being out of the way would no longer be possible, for mothers especially, once the baby arrived. For some young people, news of the pregnancy caused further breakdown in family relations and independence became necessary, even if not desired. However, for a number of reasons, independence can be more difficult to achieve and maintain when a young person has a child to consider than it is for a young person without a child.

In their move to independence, young single parents often miss a transitional period when young people first leave home or are forced to leave home and can 'practise' independence. That is not to say that independence is any less permanent or important to many young people without children. Clearly many have no more chance of returning to the family home, if there is one, than do many young parents. However, unencumbered by a child, most young people have a degree of flexibility in how they approach their first independence. For example, many young single people leave home and stay in a number of different places: with friends, cohabiting temporarily or permanently with a partner, in student accommodation, or sharing accommodation with several others. Whilst not ideal in many cases, these first, and often brief or temporary attempts at independence need not have long-term detrimental effects and to a certain extent are what society expects. However, that flexibility in type and length of accommodation is not acceptable for a young woman with a child, and indeed would be considered inappropriate by social and health services or those with a responsibility for child protection.

Perhaps the key issue here is the term 'accommodation'. Society does not expect a young person to leave the family home and immediately set up another long-term home, and neither do many young people, as much of this volume illustrates. A young mother on the other hand is expected to establish a stable and permanent home for herself and her baby on leaving the family home, care or a hostel. This mother told of the difficulty: *If I could have got it right, like a real home right away . . . it didn't have no curtains and it were cold and just horrible to be there.* A young single mother has then, not necessarily any greater need for safe, secure accommodation but a greater need for long-term stable housing in its broadest sense. That is to say, she needs more permanent accommodation in which to develop a secure long-term home, and from which she and her child will put down roots and establish themselves as a household within a community.

The transition to independence for young single parents is made more difficult because it must coincide with transition to maturity, responsibility and adulthood, often beyond their years (Clark and Coleman 1991). This situation need not necessarily be the case for a single non-parent. An added strain is placed on the parents to calculate household budgets more precisely, not to be without heat and light, and basically not to mismanage any area of life. Rather, to spin all plates – housing, budgets, personal care and care of a child – at the same time. No one area can be sacrificed for a few days to compensate for mismanagement or unforeseen problems. This greater responsibility, however, must often be handled without greater support or financial help, especially for teenaged parents.

Given their need to care for children and their young age, often coupled with limited employment experience, young parents are more likely than their non-parent peers to be dependent on welfare benefits. Whilst Income Support of £61.45 per week for a single mother aged 18 is higher than the £39.85 a non-parent would receive at the same age, the benefit has to pay for the heating, furnishing and maintenance of a family home rather than for single person's accommodation. The benefit has also, obviously, got to feed and clothe a child. This added financial stress is often the cause of young single mothers abandoning their tenancies. One teenage mother told of the difficulties which caused her to give up her flat: *It were everything really, the flat, the bairn, the money . . . Couldn't make ends meet, don't know how anyone can.* Housing Benefit for a young single mother is not restricted to the amount for shared accommodation, as it would be for a young non-parent. However, as will be discussed later, help with housing costs still presents problems and limits the housing choices for some.

HOUSING TYPE AND TENURE RESTRICTIONS

Young parents' housing choices are constrained by their need for family housing, and this in turn restricts many young parents to rented accommodation. Unlike their non-parent peers who may require only a minimum size of accommodation and limited facilities, a young parent requires two bedrooms and private kitchen and bathroom facilities. These needs immediately exclude them from many single persons' housing projects or from houses of multiple occupancy (HMOs). Young parents need a housing environment which is in all ways suitable for raising children, and from which they can gain access to a range of services such as schools, nurseries or clinics, which their non-parent peers do not need. Young parents also generally require or desire longer-term tenancies than a non-parent might. As Rugg (this volume) has shown, a long tenancy is not necessarily important to young non-parents.

Young single parents' dependence on benefits and their often urgent need for family housing confines them to the rented sector. Owner occupation amongst never-married mothers of all ages, at around 6 per cent, is so limited as not to warrant discussion here. Young parents are, therefore, limited to family housing within the diminishing local authority sector, housing association or private rented property. The avenue which offers the greatest chance of long-term success and stability depends on a number of factors, including the mother's age, the amount of property in different sectors, the level of support and degree of inter-agency working in the authority around family support issues.

Local authority

The route to local authority property is either via a housing register or via homelessness. Application for a property under homelessness legislation may have different results depending on the authority, and it is by no means the case that a young single woman with a child would be housed any more quickly than any other family with dependent children. Authorities with little available stock may require a mother to go into homeless person's accommodation prior to being offered a property. The effect of the move depends on the type of accommodation and the support services attached to it. Some authorities place young mothers with babies in their existing homeless families hostels or in bed and breakfast accommodation, whilst others have more suitable accommodation specifically for young mothers. For example, Wansbeck District Council has a hostel specifically for single mothers and babies. Within such an environment a young mother is likely to receive specialist advice and support, both with her new parenting if necessary and with her future housing decisions, and is more likely to be able to make informed decisions about her first independent housing. Some authorities make use of voluntary organisations, such as Catholic Care or the Girls' Friendly Society, to provide mother and baby hostels, although this is more often the case for those mothers for whom social services are in the process of conducting a review for child protection purposes.

Part VII of the Housing Act 1996 placed a duty on the local housing authority to secure accommodation for at least two years for those who are unintentionally homeless and from a priority need group, which includes pregnant women and families with dependent children. However, there is potential for problems where a mother is deemed to be intentionally homeless, particularly when the mother is 16 or 17 years of age. There was some confusion in the early 1990s as to which agency had final responsibility to house an intentionally homeless mother and child under the terms of the 1989 Children Act. A number of situations came to light where mothers had been passed back and forth between housing and social services, each claiming her housing was the responsibility of the other. In 1994 the duty was ultimately reaffirmed as lying with the social services departments. The situation has further improved following the election of the Labour government. The new regulations brought into effect from 1 November 1997 mean that those to whom the local authority owe a duty under homelessness legislation should also be given 'reasonable preference' in the allocation of longer-term social tenancies through the housing register. This recognition of the importance of some degree of security and longer-term accommodation may have more significance to a young single mother trying to settle into a community and establish support networks, than to a non-parent peer.

With an obligation to house the vulnerable or priority homeless quickly, a local authority with vacant property – such as Newcastle upon Tyne City Council – will offer a young mother the first available property. However, available property is likely to be in an area of high turnover and be difficult to let. The number of offers a young mother may receive differs between authorities, but many will make no more than two offers. The mother may only refuse a property if she can prove it to be unsuitable. However, few young women, faced with a longer time in B&B or homeless persons' accommodation and eager to establish homes with their children, are likely to be able to argue the suitability of a property. A young non-parent may be able to hold out for a better offer.

If not presenting as homeless, a young mother is unlikely to be awarded points simply because she is a young mother. As with any other applicant, her current housing situation will be taken into account, along with the availability of the type of family property she needs. If she is living with her parents but not living in overcrowded conditions, and is not in an unsafe situation or threatened with homelessness, she will not receive any priority points. Ironically, in Newcastle upon Tyne, where there is a surplus of one- or two-bedroomed flats in tower blocks and where there is a policy of not letting high-rise flats to families with children, the allocations system and availability favours single non-parents.

There is evidence to suggest that any delay in being housed, during which single mothers may be staying in the parental home with their babies, could put a strain on the family, especially if there are younger siblings at home (Speak *et al.* 1995). It is interesting to note that many of those housed via the homelessness route had been on the waiting list for some time prior to being housed as homeless. What may be criticised by some as the engineering of homeless status, may in fact be a realistic move to assure family relations remain intact, as this mother commented:

> *They* [the housing department] *weren't doing owt. I'd been wait-ing months, over a year and there wasn't room like, not really 'cause me and Jenny* [sister] *shared so then there was three of us with the baby. In the end my mam said they'd have to give me a place 'cause it were getting her down well and me dad. So she wrote and told them that I couldn't stay no longer, that she'd turn me out. I don't think she would have liken not really.*

Faced with such a long wait, or property in a poor location, some mothers look to other housing solutions. In 1996/7, 7.5 per cent of all lettings to housing association properties were to single parents aged between 16 and 25 (Pleace *et al.* 1998). Although housing asso-ciations often target their lettings for specific groups such as lone parents, this type of specialist provision can be patchy and supply in a given area is not always guaranteed.

Private rented housing

During the 1970s both the Finer Committee and the Housing Advisory Group expressed concern about the number of lone parent families in private rented property, especially furnished property. These concerns centred on worries about security of tenure, and safety and quality of both the property and the furnish-ings and fittings it contained. Conversely, recent governments have urged local authorities in their enabling role to make greater use of the private rented sector, suggesting that people 'should endeavour to meet their own needs' rather than expect the state to provide housing for them (Department of the Environment 1994). Faced with long waits or property in difficult-to-let areas, many young mothers do endeavour to meet their own needs and seek pri-vate rented property. However, the enabling role of a local housing authority proved little help to this mother: *All they* [the local housing office] *did was send me to an advice centre. They weren't much help, just gave me a list of private landlords . . . just left me to find a place on my own. They were no help really.*

There are a number of issues associated with private rented property which potentially present greater problems for young single mothers than for their non-parent peers. Availability is limited in many parts of the country, and to choose this tenure may well mean moving to another area or part of town, so leaving vital family support systems which are arguably more important for young parents. Availability for young mothers is limited still further by the fact that a mother needs family accommodation, rather than the bedsit, studio, or shared accommodation which her non-parent peers may find perfectly suitable. In many parts of the country, landlords are able to get better returns for turning family houses into one-person flats or multiple occupancy dwellings more suitable for single non-parents. The result is greater demand and increased rents for the remaining suitable family property. The rent for some of the suitable family property in good areas is now higher than Housing Benefit will pay. Even if the rent is affordable many landlords will not accept tenants on benefit because of the length of time it takes to process benefit claims. Many, if not most, will also require a deposit of possibly one month's rent in advance and a bond to hold against damage to the property. Whilst this situation applies to non-parents as well as parents, the amounts of money involved are greater in the case of the parent, simply because of the higher rents for family property. For example in Newcastle upon Tyne, a bond and a month's rent can amount to over £800 in order to access an ordinary two-bedroom flat. Housing Benefit payments will not cover either of these costs before the start of a tenancy, although in cases of extreme need social services have been known to help with a deposit for single mothers, and the Social Fund may offer a loan to cover rent in advance.

Young mothers desperately trying to set up an independent home, but facing difficulties finding a bond or deposit, may well be pushed towards private property in the lower end of the market. Some private landlords of lower quality properties may be willing to accept young tenants with children and on Housing Benefit and may not ask for a bond or deposit. However, they may be less than reliable at spending money on repairs and the statutory safety checks required. Moreover, as this mother explains, the legal status of the tenancy may be in doubt: [He] *just said as long as I paid my rent and didn't make any trouble I could stay, didn't have to sign anything, no.* As this example indicates, another problem associated with private rented property is security of tenure. Most young parents are hoping to settle into a long-term stable housing situation very quickly and do not wish to move for many years. In this respect young mothers do not see private renting, with six- or twelve-month tenancies, as secure.

This review of the issues relating to different tenures for single young parents must be taken in the context of changing housing situations across the country, and the acceptance of the diminution of all local authority stock and the state of the local private rented market. It ·is fair to say that whilst single young mothers may prefer a particular tenure, they may have no option but to take what is available. The extent to which a young mother's desire to leave home, or the urgency of her need to leave, is affected by the supply of available property in different tenures in the area is questionable. There is little doubt that most young single mothers do want to establish themselves in an independent home as soon as possible, but to achieve this there are considerable barriers to overcome. However, the problems they experience once independently housed are often greater than the problems of getting initial housing. These problems will be discussed later in the chapter.

WHAT ABOUT FATHERS?

Thus far this chapter has concentrated on young single mothers. However, the babies' fathers, whilst frequently perceived as being totally disassociated with their children, often do play a large part in their care, much as any other separated father might (Burghes et al. 1997; Ruxton and Burgess 1996; Speak et al. 1997). Housing is important to any young man trying to establish independence, but for a father it can play a central role in allowing him to maintain a relationship with his child and support the mother, even after their relationship has ended. However, young single fathers are not part of the priority need group under Part VII of the 1996 Housing Act, and are often seen as problematic rather than vulnerable. Therefore they are generally a very low priority for any available social housing. Furthermore, classed as single, rather than as a family as the mothers and children are, the young fathers are subject to the Single Room Rent restrictions in Housing Benefit payments which means that they are unlikely to be able to afford accommodation in which it is suitable for a baby or young child to sleep over (Rugg, this volume).

Estranged fathers, whether young or older, single, separated or divorced, often express a desire for suitable family housing from which to offer their children a 'second home'. However, both their low priority status for social housing and the Single Room Rent mean that many find this impossible (Simpson et al. 1995; Speak et al. 1997). Asked what he felt would help his relationship with his child one young man commented: *a place of my own, with a room just for him like, so he'd know he had a home another one and . . . it was there for him . . . like he had two homes.* Another young man who remained in the family home felt the pressure to move once he had his child to stay and it was no longer suitable for him to share a room with his brother. He explained what had made him decide to get his own place: *Our Kevin come in pissed, well served* [drunk] *he was . . . I said to him you have to be quiet and that with babies but he were too pissed to listen. I said to him next day and he were sorry like.* In some cities where there is a surplus of property on the larger local authority estates young single men can be housed quite quickly. Other young men resort to renting privately. In both cases, the quality of the property or neighbourhood may be less than suitable for a child, even temporarily.

PROBLEMS WITH FIRST INDEPENDENT HOUSING

Few young single parents make the transition to independence without a number of problems. Their young age and lack of experience make even small problems associated with housing difficult to manage. Young parents are more restricted in their mobility than other young people. They not only suffer from extreme poverty but their freedom and social lives are further constrained by their parenthood. Many spend long, often lonely, hours in isolation trying to entertain themselves and their children in their immediate home and environment. Their home and neighbourhood can become their world. Moreover, many young parents are unaware of the unsuitability of the property or area until after they move in, at which point they are effectively trapped: because they are no longer homeless, or threatened with homelessness, the young parent will be seen by the authority as suitably housed. This mother commented on her hasty decision to accept a property which proved to be unsuitable:

It were damp and there were cockroaches. It was disgusting. I told them but they just said 'you accepted it'. Honest, it weren't fit for a dog, let alone a bairn. And all round the windows was rotten so the rain came in.

It is not only young mothers who suffer from unsuitable property in poor locations. Young fathers too, trying to take some responsibility for the care of their children, have commented on the unsuitability of their local authority property.

> *I could have her* [daughter] *back at my place but I don't like . . . not overnight, I mean not my place, I mean it's too rough for a little lass . . . aye, they're drunk, pissed and doing drugs and that there's mostly trouble mostly every night like, well, at the weekends when I have her . . . it's not right for a little lass.*

This father's comments highlight another aspect particularly associated with local authority property which causes concern to many young parents. In many cases it is not the quality of the property which is inadequate, but the neighbourhood in which it is situated. A number of studies have claimed that not only do lone parents tend to end up in the least desirable types of housing but also in the least desirable areas of council accommodation, and studies of younger parents reaffirm this finding (Finer 1974; Hardy and Crow 1991; Kahn and Henderson 1987).

Like other parents, the majority of young single parents are acutely aware of the effects of their environment on their children. Whilst most make pleasant and comfortable homes for their families within the confines of the flat or house, they are unable to control the adverse affects of the neighbourhood: as one interviewee commented: *Can't let him play out, not round here, with the swearing and that.* Vandalism, misuse of the neighbourhood, such as rubbish tipping and the activities of gangs of youths, or fear of crime and harassment are all issues which make living difficult on some of the social housing estates where most young single parents find themselves housed:

> *You can see them* [youths] *. . . all at the back of the garages at night. They're sniffing like . . . and other stuff. They don't even try to hide it, you can see the bags and things in the morning. The bairns pick stuff up. I've reported it but they didn't do nowt.*

Unfortunately, once housed, rehousing or a transfer may be very difficult. However unsuitable the property or area, with a child to house and support, mothers particularly do not have the freedom to leave until they have secured alternative accommodation. Without a child to consider, a single young person could leave and stay with friends or relatives until something better could be found, or at least spend as little time as possible in the offending property. In some cases, of course, the existence of a child may make friends or relatives more likely to take a single young person in, for the sake of the child. The young woman commenting below had spent several months living in unsuitable property and trying to get rehoused. The property she was offered was in an even more unsuitable location for her child so she had to return to her family. Not all young parents are lucky enough to be able to do this:

> *They said I could have a house down the bottom* [of the estate]. *It were next to the* **** [a family known for their criminal activity]. *I wasn't going to bring up a bairn next to them like. I had to go back to my mam's and wait. It took two years.*

Even if the neighbourhood proves suitable, the housing a new mother with a baby needs initially may be very different to the housing she needs a few years later when her child is beginning to grow or starts school. In the first stages of independence, a mother's priority may be to be near her family for support. This need may well override all other considerations and lead her to accept property in a condition, or in an area, which is not suitable for the longer term. As she becomes more confident and her child grows she may find she needs less family support but larger or better accommodation, perhaps a garden too. Once her child can play out and has friends a range of factors which would not affect a non-parent may become relevant, such as the location of schools or playgrounds or the quality of the neighbourhood However, unless she is awarded points for ill health, overcrowding or harassment, rehousing can present greater problems than initial housing, as she will be considered adequately housed and therefore no longer be seen as a priority. As one mother commented:

> *I'm on the list like but I don't know how long it will take. It's shocking round here now. Never used to be like this when I were a kid. It were OK then. I can't take much more, daren't hardly go out of my house.*

In such situations some mothers suffer physical or mental ill health caused by the stress of their living conditions. In Newcastle upon

Tyne in 1993/4 over 10 per cent of the mothers who were rehoused under the local authority transfer system had medical priority points. The main reason given for the points was depression stemming from the social problems of the neighbourhood.

A house is not a home

The material comforts needed to turn a house into a home suitable for a baby or small child are arguably greater than those needed for a single person. Moreover, a mother needs to achieve certain standards quickly. Whilst a couple or single person without children could take time to accumulate furniture or domestic equipment, a young mother needs certain items immediately. A refrigerator for food hygiene, carpets to save small knees from splinters and to keep the home warm, and a washing machine for the large amount of washing and drying that a small child generates are not luxuries but necessities. Many young mothers, though, live extremely impoverished lives once they are in their own homes and have to go without even the most basic of home furnishings and comforts for several years.

The Social Fund, set up to provide grants and loans for people in need, has been well reported on in recent years (Craig 1993; Huby and Dix 1992; NACAB 1990). Predominantly the Social Fund offers loans, rather than grants: only those re-establishing themselves in the community from a care situation would receive a grant. In this respect, the Fund does not favour young parents over young non-parents. A young single mother claiming benefits may be able to get a loan to buy basic household furnishings and equipment, but she will have to repay the loan from her limited Income Support. A young father would almost certainly not be able to get help from the Social Fund to equip a home for a visiting child.

Many authorities are now offering furnished lettings or providing furniture packs through voluntary agencies (Rooney 1997). The quality of the goods varies greatly from place to place, but in general the help this provides is extremely valuable in the early days of independence. Furthermore, a furnished tenancy limits the need for credit and debt which plague so many young mothers, and which cannot be accommodated by Income Support. Young fathers, however, although often also eligible for assistance of this kind, would generally only receive furniture for a single person.

Additional items needed to provide suitable accommodation for a visiting child would not be provided.

Issues of support

The main form of support to most young single mothers is family. The need to remain near their families is one of the main reasons young mothers find it so difficult to be suitably housed, and one of the reasons so many do continue to live with their parents for as long as possible in the hope that a local authority property in the right area will become available. Regardless of the tenure chosen, many find they have to move to other parts of the town or city to get independent accommodation, thus breaking valuable support networks. On Income Support, few can afford costly bus fares, and this exacerbates their isolation. Distance from family and support networks is also problematic for single fathers living independently of their families. Those who are trying to establish or maintain relationships with their children or their children's mothers, whilst not cohabiting with them or after the relationships with the mothers have ended, need more support than fathers who are not trying to maintain relationships. One young man, housed at the opposite side of the city to the neighbourhood where he had grown up, told this tale of his first independence:

> It were fine, a good flat and a good size . . . but I felt right out of it, 'cause I've grown up here [in a west end neighbourhood of Newcastle upon Tyne] all my life and my mates are here and K and C [his son and the child's mother] only live round the corner, and I hardly saw them.

Another young single father commented: I could go all day, more and not see no one. Yeh, I were lonely, I suppose.

Young single fathers may need to be housed near their families to receive support, but also in order to give support. Because little is known about the situation surrounding young single fatherhood, it is difficult to say how many young fathers are actively involved in the raising of their children. The Fatherhood Study was based on the assumption that a percentage do wish to be involved, that such involvement should be encouraged, and that fathers may face a range of barriers to that involvement. Housing was shown to be one such barrier. Many of the fathers in the Fatherhood Study were keen to help in the daily care of their children. Often they provided a valuable form of support for the mothers as one young man explained: *K* [the child's mother] *gets depression . . . I think she'd find it too hard* [without my help]. *At least I can take our L* [daughter] *out and give her a break.* This father, like many others, was involved on a daily basis with the care of his child, which would not have been possible had he lived further away. Other fathers offered support and baby sitting to allow the mothers to go out to work or to attend training courses.

CONCLUSION

Clearly single young parents have different housing needs to young single non-parents in terms of the size, quality and location of their homes. They are also the poorest of young people, with a greater dependence on state benefits and the least able to take part-time work to supplement their incomes. These young people are therefore limited to renting the cheapest housing available in any sector, being unlikely to be able to afford any shortfall between Housing Benefit and rent. Thus there is a greater likelihood that they will have a more socially and materially impoverished start to their independent lives than most young people. Moreover, their children are more likely to begin their lives in poverty. Because of their potentially long-term dependence on welfare benefits, this impoverishment is likely to be long lived and difficult to overcome. As a consequence, the children of young single parents, whilst receiving as much care and love as any other children, often begin, and continue, their lives at a disadvantage. Poor housing is just one of the ways in which that disadvantage manifests itself, but poor housing and the issues associated with it, as discussed here in relation to both mothers and fathers, have a knock-on effect on other aspects of life.

Housing is just one part of a complex process which these young parents are undertaking. The mothers especially had very little flexibility in their approach to gaining and maintaining independent housing, and it is this lack of flexibility which made their housing situation impinge so much on other parts of the processes they were engaged in – growing up, learning to care for themselves and a child, learning to manage budgets and often coping with the end of a relationship. Current housing policy and practice does not recognise the role of housing in this wider process. Moreover, current policy is often counter-productive in relation to the objectives of other government policies. For example, young single fathers are being pursued by the Child Support Agency for maintenance, which many cannot pay because of their poor position in the labour market. At the same time both lone parents and young people in general are being made the focus of attention on unemployment through such policies as the New Deal (Speak 1998). However, for those who are both lone parents and young unemployed people, housing has a crucial role to play in their ability to get and keep a job. For example, it seems likely that more young single fathers, particularly those with time on their hands because of unemployment, are prepared to take responsibility for the care of their children than is normally assumed. It is also becoming clear that young mothers both want to work and are in a better position to get work in the new services sector jobs, but find affordable childcare the biggest barrier (Marsh and McKay 1993). Housing policy could have a role in bringing mother and father together in a mutually convenient way. By recognising that some young single fathers need family housing for their children, housing policy could assist them to provide childcare, allowing young mothers to come off benefits. In this respect, rather than being one of the problems produced as the result of changing family formation, housing could be central to the solution.

All young people need a high degree of flexibility in their early independent lives, both with regard to housing and employment, as they learn to prioritise different areas of life. However, young parents, who arguably need the most flexibility if they are to negotiate the best situation for their young families, have limited choice. Youth is a time for learning, experimenting and making mistakes. One of the most important factors affecting housing for young parents is the fact that they are deprived of this crucial learning time. Mistakes, though, are still made, but they have a more disruptive and longer-term effect. Many policies, including housing policies, do not acknowledge the importance of this transitional stage in life for young people. Furthermore, policies are increasingly designed to encourage a level of uniform behaviour, as if young people were a homogeneous group. This sub-group of young single parents highlights the error of this assumption. Moreover, policies increasingly also fail to offer a safety net for the difficulties which many young people naturally encounter. Housing policies in particular are increasingly based on the assumption that young people can and should remain with their families until they are able to support themselves financially, and that they can turn to their families for support in the event of a problem. For many young single parents, both mothers and fathers, it is their status as parents which is perceived as a problem, which makes relying on family less feasible and to succeed independently more important.

Chapter 10

No cardboard boxes, so no problem?

Young people and housing in rural areas

Anwen Jones

A fifth of young people between the ages of 16 and 24 in England live in rural areas, yet most research on youth issues and the problems facing young people has tended to focus on urban youth. In rural housing research, as Burrows *et al.* (1998) note, there has been a tendency to simply 'tag on' consideration of young people to existing studies. Where rural youth housing issues have been addressed these have usually examined the most extreme form of housing need, homelessness. This chapter describes the rural housing problem and goes on to examine the housing difficulties faced specifically by young people in rural areas. The chapter draws on a recent study by Ford *et al.* (1997) of young people and housing in rural areas, and ongoing research by Jones and Rugg on the housing and labour market experiences of young people in rural North Yorkshire.[1] Changes in housing and welfare policies and their consequences for young people have been discussed elsewhere (Anderson, Rugg, this volume) and are therefore only briefly referred to here. However, some attention is paid to those specific policies which have had an impact on the rural housing situation. It is suggested that the problems facing young people in rural areas are not dissimilar to those facing their urban counterparts, but may be exacerbated by aspects of rurality. A number of structural factors need to be addressed in order for young people to have a real choice about whether to leave or to stay in the country-side. However, there is also a need for further research which examines the expectations of young people and how these are shaped by structural factors over which they have little control.

THE RURAL HOUSING PROBLEM

In recent years there has been growing recognition of the significant and in some ways distinctive rural housing problem. In particular, a shortage of affordable housing has been seen by the Rural Development Commission (RDC) as one of the most important issues facing rural communities (RDC 1993). A growing body of research identifies a number of key points as central to the rural housing problem: both demand and supply influences have been recognised as having an impact on the availability of housing.

At a very basic level there are two forms of demand in rural areas: that which is generated by the existing population and that which comes from outside the area (Shucksmith *et al.* 1995). Most areas will have demand for housing from the local population, but some will also experience additional pressure from outside their community. Competition for housing is heightened by demand for second homes, homes for retirement migrants, and long-distance commuters (Robinson 1992). Migration to rural areas is prompted by a variety of motives; for example, housing-related reasons and a desire for rural life (A. E. Green 1997). As well as those who choose to live in the countryside there are those who, to some extent, are constrained into doing so because they cannot afford urban prices. Given the differences between the two groups as to motive and income, Shucksmith *et al.* (1995) suggest that they are unlikely to move into the same areas or to compete for the same type of property. Both groups, however, will have the effect of increasing demand in an area and thereby pushing prices up. As more urban dwellers move into the countryside or purchase second homes there, long-term rural residents and their children find it more difficult to secure suitable and affordable accommodation. This is the 'no homes for locals' issue, which is considered by one commentator to be 'one of the most alarming and emotive problems of a number of difficulties that can be considered under the umbrella of rural housing problems' (Robinson 1992: 111).

There are difficulties associated with measuring the level of housing demand as secondary data sources only allow analysis of expressed demand – such as joining a housing register or forming a new household (Shucksmith *et al.* 1995). The data do not allow for the assessment of latent demand – for example from young people who may wish to live independently but remain in the

parental home because they cannot afford to move out. Cloke *et al.*
(1995) also make the point that there have been considerable differences of opinion over both the level of housing need in rural areas
and the best way to respond to identified need. Nevertheless, qualitative evidence from Cloke *et al.*'s (1994) study suggests that housing
need can be presumed to exist in most areas and that these needs are
being reproduced over time.

In 1990 it was estimated that 377,100 rural households were
specifically in housing need, while house prices in rural areas
were 10–15 per cent above the national average (Simmons 1997).
A study carried out by the RDC in 1990 concluded that there was
a net requirement of at least 80,000 additional homes in rural
England over the following five years: approximately 16,000
homes a year. By 1993 only about 8,800 affordable homes for rent
or shared ownership had been built, just 11 per cent of the RDC's
estimated need (RDC 1993). The most obvious and extreme indicator of housing need is homelessness and in 1992 the RDC found
that homelessness in deeply rural areas had tripled in four years
compared to a doubling in urban areas (RDC 1993). As the population of rural areas continues to grow, as does the number of households, the need for affordable housing will remain high.

On the supply side there are a number of significant factors which
have an impact on the availability and affordability of housing
in addition to competition from higher income groups. Planning
policies limit the supply of new housing by restricting the availability
of land as well as increasing the cost of building. Over 30 per cent of
rural England is designated as National Park, Area of Outstanding
Beauty or Green Belt and much of the remainder is subject to a
presumption against development. Rural housing schemes are also
more expensive to build because of high land costs and the higher
unit costs of building small sites often in remote areas (Kilburn
1996). Planning constraints designed to help retain local character
add to the cost of rural housing by specifying the use of vernacular
materials. There is some evidence that these cost and planning pressures are causing developments to be skewed towards market towns
and large villages, despite the high level of need in small villages
(RDC 1993).

HOUSING YOUNG PEOPLE IN RURAL AREAS

The incidence of housing need is a well-established fact of orthodox accounts of the rural housing problem. However, as in the literature on rural deprivation and housing generally, little attention has been given to the specific needs of young people. Many chapters in this volume indicate that young people face multiple obstacles when attempting to secure accommodation in every tenure: the nature of the rural housing problem can exacerbate these difficulties for young people hoping to continue living in the countryside.

Ford (this volume) has indicated that young people are now less likely to enter into owner occupation. However, in the countryside this tenure has absorbed a higher proportion of the housing stock: 75 per cent of dwellings are in owner occupation in rural areas, compared with 64 per cent in urban areas (DoE and MAFF 1995). Even aside from a general unwillingness to enter owner occupation, the nature of the rural housing stock is such that there may be little in the way of affordable or appropriate owner occupation for first time entrants. Detached houses and bungalows constitute over 40 per cent of the rural housing stock, compared with only about 15 per cent of urban housing stock. Semi-detached houses are also significantly over-represented in rural areas, whilst terraced houses and flats – the type of properties which are generally cheaper and sought by first time buyers – are significantly under-represented. Traditionally those who cannot afford to buy have looked to the rented sector for accommodation. Again there are differences between rural and urban areas which have a significant impact on young people's prospects in the housing market.

Social housing is under-represented in rural areas. In urban areas, social housing and housing association accommodation houses over 24 per cent of households whilst in rural areas this sector houses just over 15 per cent (Ford *et al.* 1997). In contrast to the national situation where, since the First World War, public sector housing has grown to compensate for the decline in private rented accommodation, the social sector has never been a major component in the rural housing stock. Furthermore, the distribution of this limited social housing has been uneven, reflecting the impact of housing policies, the pattern of physical infrastructure and local authority housing investment decisions. McLaughlin (1986) found several parishes where there was no social housing at all. The situation has been exacerbated by the Right to Buy policy, especially as the take-up of this opportunity by existing tenants has been greater in rural areas where council housing has been relatively more attractive. For the same reason the rate of turnover (relets) in the remaining local authority stock has been relatively low so that few properties become available for new tenants.

The difficulties which stem from the limited availability of housing are exacerbated by the processes whereby social housing is obtained or allocated (Anderson, this volume). Button cites a National Children's Home survey, which found evidence of more restrictive practices being applied in rural areas that prevented young people from gaining access to council housing (Button 1992). Anderson (1997) found that housing associations were more sensitive to the needs of young people; but, until recently, most housing association investment was concentrated in urban areas (Bramley and Smart 1995; Bevan and Sanderling 1996). Young people living in rural areas who cannot afford to compete in the owner occupied sector and who are denied access to social housing have, like young people elsewhere, often no alternative but to look for private rented accommodation.

The private rented sector houses one in ten of all households in England but one in eight in rural areas (Rhodes and Bevan 1997). The increased significance of the sector in the countryside is reflected in the fact that the Conservative government aimed to improve access to affordable housing in rural areas by encouraging expansion within the private sector (Bevan and Sanderling 1996). The government also considered the private sector as being particularly suitable for meeting demand for housing from under-25s. However, commentators have argued that for young people on relatively low incomes and not always in need of the self-contained family housing the rural rented sector offers, private renting is often unsuitable and financially out of their reach (Button 1992). Button cites RDC research on homelessness which suggests that the rural private rented sector is relatively insignificant as a source of permanent low-cost accommodation (Button 1992).

There are a number of reasons why reliance on the rural private rented sector for young people's housing remains problematic. Reports have described the general difficulties faced by young people in their attempts to secure access to private renting (Rugg 1996, 1997), but features of the rural sector exacerbate these problems. For example, higher rental charges have knock-on effects on the requirement to pay a higher amount of rent in advance, and a deposit usually equivalent to a month's rent. Research has shown that private landlords least preferred to let to young people and unemployed people (Crook and Kemp 1996), and demand for rural property can be so high that landlords are in a position to exercise some degree of choice over the type of tenant to which they prefer to let (Bevan and Sanderling 1996). Indeed, analysis of census data found that a smaller proportion of single persons were private renting in rural areas than in urban areas (Bevan and Sanderling 1996). The nature of the rural private rented sector further disadvantages young people. While the size of the private rented sector appears proportionately larger than in urban areas, some of it is tied accommodation and not always available to the young (Ford *et al.* 1997). Bevan and Sanderling (1996) found that almost 90 per cent of privately rented accommodation was composed of houses. A much smaller proportion was composed of flats than was the case in urban areas. In addition, nearly three-quarters of furnished privately rented dwellings – a type of let most suitable for young people – consisted of houses. Almost all privately rented accommodation in rural areas was self-contained and 96 per cent of renting households in rural areas were in dwellings with three or more bedrooms. Only 1 per cent were living in bedsits compared with 11 per cent living in bedsits in urban areas. The limited availability of housing suitable for shared arrangements has serious consequences for young people reliant on Housing Benefit to meet rental costs, since assistance will not cover the higher rents charged by landlords for self-contained accommodation (Rugg, this volume).

One of the most important structural factors influencing young people's housing circumstances are the local labour market opportunities, but other aspects of rurality combine to further disadvantage young people in rural areas. For Shucksmith *et al.* (1995) the basic requirement for enjoying free choice of where to live is having the money to afford housing and transport. Donnison agrees, suggesting that most housing problems are really problems of unemployment, poverty and inequality (Hutson and Liddiard 1994). Many features of the rural youth labour market are recognisable in urban contexts, but there are also distinctive rural aspects such as the predominance of small firms, lack of access to training and lower than average wage rates (Turbin and Stern 1987). Rural labour markets are no more homogeneous than their urban counterparts and the employment opportunities open to young people vary with the degree of access to urban centres of employment. Transport, as suggested above, is extremely important and can place constraints on both the housing and employment opportunities open to young people. A RDC study (1994a) found that 73 per cent of parishes had no daily bus service. In some areas, where public transport does exist, buses may run only twice a day and in some cases only once or twice a week. In rural areas with such a limited transport infrastructure private transport is often a necessity. Even with some private transport the numbers and jobs available in rural areas present very difficult problems for young people (Cloke *et al.* 1994). It is widely recognised that the lack of opportunity in local labour and housing markets has led to the out-migration of many young people, who may be obliged to leave for their education, jobs and housing (Campbell *et al.* 1996; Cloke *et al.* 1994; Jones and Jamieson 1996; RDC 1994b).

YOUNG PEOPLE'S EXPERIENCE OF THE RURAL HOUSING MARKET

The issues discussed above give some indication of the rural housing problem, the structure and supply of rural housing and some of the difficulties facing young people. But how do young people experience the rural housing market, what are their needs and preferences, and how do structural factors shape expectations and opportunities? Work completed by Ford *et al.* (1997), and Jones and Rugg's ongoing study, draws a much more complex picture of young people in the rural housing market than simply indicating degrees of constraint. This work develops a typology of a combination of young people's experiences and expectations, and in doing so builds to some degree on the work of Dench (cited in Jones 1992), who suggests that for many young people the decision to leave rural areas is often a painful one, and that a far greater proportion of young people would remain or return to rural areas if they had a choice.

First, it must be stressed that young people in the countryside do not have a uniform experience of rural housing problems, basically because rural housing markets are not homogeneous. Although the structure of provision is broadly similar and the pressure and sources of demand vary, Shucksmith *et al.* (1995) have been able to classify six types of rural housing market using a range of variables, integrating both demand- and supply-side influences. For example, their analysis recognises rural housing markets which are characterised by land constraints and pressure from retirement and holiday-home buyers, as well as indigenous demand (which tend to predominate in the south and south-east of England). A second example is where the supply of land is less constrained and demand comes from retirement in-migrants and the established population. There is a low turnover of housing stock and the area may experience out-migration of young people (the wards in this category occur typically in Northumberland, Durham, North Yorkshire, Humberside, Lincolnshire, Lancashire, Cheshire and Staffordshire). Rural housing markets where land supply is constrained and demand comes from commuters and fluid populations tend to form an inner ring around London. These areas are characterised by long-distance commuting (over twenty miles), and high house prices. Residential turnover is rapid and local housing opportunities are few.

Ford *et al.* (1997) acknowledged the need to base their research on rural youth in a range of housing markets, and completed their study of young people in six different housing markets and one tourist area. They found the structure of housing provision was broadly similar in the six areas (the tourist area differed having a much larger private rented sector associated with the tourist trade): there was very limited social housing, the private rented sector was small and often very expensive and the main tenure was owner occupation. As Shucksmith *et al.* (1995) suggested, the exact nature of demand for housing varied: there was always a mix of commuters and retired people but sometimes weighted to one group more than the other. In some areas accommodation for owner occupation was more rather than less available and its price varied. However, for young people these differences were largely irrelevant: 'Nowhere could local young people compete effectively for local housing and thus the issues raised by young people about their housing needs were similar across the different housing markets' (Ford *et al.* 1997: 23). Essentially there was insufficient housing in their locality for young people and, as noted above, the problem was one of suitability and affordability.

The lack of affordable housing resulted in a range of experiences of housing need. Ford *et al.* (1997) found that need ran on a continuum from the most immediate and obvious in the form of homelessness at one end to housing need in the form of delayed entry into independent housing at the other. Rural homelessness includes those who are currently homeless in rural areas, some sleeping in holiday chalets or other temporary accommodation when there is no tourism. It also includes young people from rural areas who have become homeless in towns (Hutson and Liddiard 1994). Ford *et al.* (1997) found that there was a reluctance among some people in rural areas to admit that any housing problem existed, and anxiety about the adverse effects of such information on the tourist industry. As a YMCA project director in North Yorkshire commented:

> The greatest difficulty has been the lack of awareness from both within the community and from outsiders. The community did not want to accept that they had a homelessness problem, as it was not visible. Homelessness was about cardboard boxes. There were no cardboard boxes, so there could not be a problem.
>
> (Simmons 1997: 125)

Similarly, Ford *et al.* (1997) found, young people themselves equated homelessness with rooflessness or living in a squat, although a considerable amount of them knew people who had to move into friends' homes following conflicts with their parents. Others moved to towns where there was emergency accommodation and some help available to them. There is thus a process of exporting and urbanising homelessness and this, in part, accounts for the low homelessness rate in the very rural areas. The number of young people now living in towns and cities as a result of rural homelessness is unknown but is probably not insignificant (Ford *et al.* 1997).

At the other end of the continuum of housing need are the many young people who wish to establish independent living arrangements but are prevented from doing so by the absence of suitable and affordable accommodation. Their position reflects a different but nevertheless important form of homelessness (Burton *et al.* 1989a; Ford *et al.* 1997). The cost of housing and its relationship to young people's incomes was a central issue raised in all the discussion groups in Ford *et al.*'s (1997) study. Ford *et al.* (1997) found that more young people had thought about trying to leave home than had actually managed to do so. Ongoing research by Jones and Rugg is finding that many young people are well aware of the difficulties of securing accommodation even though they had not tried to do so themselves. They learned from the experience of friends and from advertisements for accommodation that independent living was an unrealistic ambition given their financial circumstances. Where young people had managed to secure accommodation they often found that they could not afford to sustain independent living and returned to the parental home, a common pattern among young people generally (Jones 1995b; DaVanzo and Goldscheider 1990).

However, it is evident that young people can hold a range of views on their housing situation: some are as keen to leave rural areas as others are to stay. Ford *et al.* (1997) identified four main groups of young people in terms of their preferences and expectations with respect to staying in rural areas. These four groupings reflect the interaction between personal preference and structural constraints and are characterised as: committed leavers who wish to move away and expect to do so; reluctant stayers who wish to move away but think that they will be unable to do so; reluctant leavers who would prefer to stay but think that they will be unable to do so; and finally, committed stayers who prefer to stay in the area and expect to do so. Focus group work completed as part of Ford *et al.*'s study explored these groupings in detail.

Committed leavers

Two-thirds of the young people attending the focus groups expressed a clear preference to move away, and the majority expected that they would do so. Most of these young people were either planning further or higher education elsewhere or were recent graduates seeking professional or managerial careers which would be based in urban areas. In the meantime they lived at home with their parents. This was seen as necessary but not always appropriate or satisfactory. Ongoing work by Jones and Rugg is also finding that young people are pragmatic about returning home if they do not find employment immediately after completing their studies. Many had student debts and saw home as a comfortable and relatively cheap staging post while they looked for permanent employment.

Ford *et al.* found that although eager to move away, this group also expressed a desire to return to the area in 10–15 years' time. This is also the case among young people in Jones and Rugg's ongoing study, who had moved away to large towns and cities to attend university. Rural areas were seen as the most suitable environment for raising a family, and many young people said they enjoyed the peace and quiet of the countryside. However, these young people had also enjoyed aspects of city life, particularly being close to all facilities, the regular public transport and the night-life. Those who had been brought up in isolated rural areas or where there was very limited public transport did not want their children to 'miss out' as they had as teenagers. The ideal for almost all these young people would be to live in a rural setting but accessible to an urban area. Most of these young people expressed concern about the effects of demand from commuters, tourists and retire-ment migrants on the local housing market and were aware of the problems faced by their peers who stayed in the area and could not compete with higher income groups. There was general agree-ment that a move back to the countryside would only occur when individuals were established in their careers, were financially secure and earning enough to buy a home. Such a move would almost certainly entail commuting, as few people thought they would find suitable employment in a rural area. For these young people, it appears, moving out and getting on is seen as a means to return to the countryside one day.

Reluctant stayers

The reluctant stayers in Ford *et al.*'s study tended to be less qualified and, if employed, worked in manual or agricultural work. Their reasons for wanting to leave reflected lifestyle and social issues, the absence of transport and the resulting isolation. These young people were constrained by their lack of employment experience and skills and limited financial resources. Jones and Rugg's ongoing study found that a number of young people with few or no qualifica-tions had managed to secure employment and accommodation in another area but were forced to return to the parental home as they could not afford to live independently. Some young people repeated this pattern a number of times, which resulted in periods of unemployment punctuated by spells of insecure and/or low-paid employment which made it almost impossible for them either to further their employment experience or to save enough money to make a successful move.

Reluctant leavers

As suggested earlier, many young people in Ford *et al.*'s (1997) study preferred to stay in the locality: they loved the area and the environment and enjoyed having friends and family nearby. Only half of them, however, thought it would be possible to stay. The reluctant leavers represented a range of social and economic characteristics: some were unskilled and unemployed, others were living at home after finishing higher education and some were about to leave for university. Their reasons for leaving were related to the lack of opportunities in the area in terms of employment, housing and transport: one young person commented: 'I'd like to think I'll be here in three or four years, but actually I think I'll be in Leeds with a job and a house I can afford' (Ford *et al.* 1997: 25).

Committed stayers

Committed stayers were in the minority. These young people also shared a sense of belonging to the area, but unlike the reluctant leavers most had secured paid employment and affordable (though not always good quality) housing or were content to live with their parents. The willingness of parents to house their adult children is clearly important. In Jones and Rugg's ongoing study the majority of young people who remained in their home area lived with their parents (some had returned from living independently). Some young people were happy to remain in the parental home, others were less content but appeared willing to forgo a certain amount of independence in return for the benefits of living at home. The relatively small amount of money paid for 'keep' meant that young people could afford holidays and a social life, as well as necessities such as cars; others were saving towards independent accommodation. Some of the young people living with their parents thought that paying rent was 'money down the drain' and preferred to stay at home until they were in a position to obtain a mortgage. However, as Ford *et al.* (1997) found, not all young people were happy to live at home, and conflict with parents was one of the factors that could result in committed stayers becoming reluctant leavers.

Ford *et al.* concluded that there is continuing unmet housing need among young people in rural areas and warned that failure to meet the housing needs of young people has a number of potential implications. Young people will face continued pressures to leave rural areas, and more reluctant leavers will actually leave. Second, those who wish to stay will find it more difficult to do so. Third, where young people do stay, it may be at the cost of delaying the full transition to adult independence. Fourth, young people who do stay may have to commit substantial amounts of income to obtain independent housing, increasing the risk of poverty for those on relatively low earnings.

CONCLUSION

As Burrows *et al.* (1998) note, much debate concerned with contemporary rurality is concerned with rural drift and the emphasis has often been on analysing strategies which aim to retain rural communities for local people. Although commentators are gradually recognising the particular difficulties faced by young people trying to secure accommodation in rural areas, research has begun to demonstrate that the expectations and needs of this group are by no means uniform. It is important, as Jones (1992) suggests, that policies offer real choice to young people rather than be designed to retain them in rural areas.

In conclusion some consideration should be given to the implications of the out-migration of young people. Rural populations are ageing as a result of young people moving away, and because of the influx of older retired people. These trends result in higher house prices and reduced demand for local services. One of the outcomes of these processes is that rural areas will increasingly become dominated by high income. As Stern and Turbin (1986) and Cloke *et al.* (1994) note, the relative prosperity of such areas may obscure the problems of low income groups and young people and deter local councils and organisations from tackling certain problems relating to transport and job opportunities which would address the roots of the problems faced by young people with respect to housing (Ford *et al.* 1997). These processes will compound the problems faced by young people and result in even fewer opportunities for them to live and work in rural areas.

NOTE

1 Anwen Jones and Julie Rugg are currently undertaking a research project funded by the Joseph Rowntree Foundation entitled 'Getting a job, finding a home: capturing the dynamic of the rural youth transition'. The study, based on interviews with 60 young people living in rural North Yorkshire, will be completed by Easter 1999.

Chapter 11

Young adults living in the parental home

The implications of extended youth transitions for housing and social policy

Bob Coles, Julie Rugg and Jenny Seavers

Many chapters in this book have indicated the difficulties faced by young people trying to secure independent accommodation. A range of economic, social and housing policy obstacles hinder young people's access to home ownership, social housing and private renting. Furthermore, particular problems faced by sub-groups within the 16–25 age range can exacerbate the process of marginalisation within the main housing sectors. One common theme predominates: the increased resort by young people to accommodation in the parental home. The inability to take any first steps in their housing career means that many young people remain in the parental home for longer periods, and difficulty in sustaining tenancies and independent living again means a greater reliance on the parental home when these fail.

However, consideration of young people's housing careers should not take place in a vacuum: housing choices are made alongside employment decisions and the steps young people take to form households and families of their own. In this regard, it is appropriate to consider young people living in the parental home in the context of broader literature relating to the transitions that young people make to adult status. It has been recognised that it is increasingly difficult for young people to achieve what has been termed 'traditional' transitions between child-dependency status and full adulthood, and commentators now discuss the growth of extended and fractured transitions. Young people are facing a number of obstacles in the process of achieving independence, and beyond the housing issues outlined in some chapters in this book a number of other socio-economic factors can be associated with a longer stay in the parental home. It cannot be assumed, however, that young people living in the parental home are a homogeneous group. The limited research which does exist on this area suggests that those young people continuing to live at home do so for a variety of very different reasons, so raising a whole series of research issues. Indeed, focusing attention on the implications of young people continuing to live in the parental home for extended periods points to the need for a distinct research agenda producing material to underpin in a more informed manner policy relating to the housing needs of young people.

This chapter begins by introducing literature which outlines the changing pattern of youth transitions. Factors associated with the growth of extended transitions are examined, and particular attention is paid to their impact on family relationships. Detailed exploration then takes place of the sub-groupings of young people who continue to live in the parental home. The chapter concludes with discussion of some of the social and housing policy consequences of a heavy reliance on the parental home to house young people.

CHANGING PATTERNS OF YOUTH TRANSITIONS

Traditional, extended and fractured transitions

Within the research context, youth is often defined as a series of interrelated transitions between childhood dependency and adult citizenship. Research is often based on the conceptualisation of 'traditional transitions' and how these have been transformed by socio-economic change in the 1970s and 1980s. Traditional transitions were defined as largely linear sequences of statuses whereby young people left school at minimum school leaving age and found work, saved, formed relationships, married, and upon marriage moved away from the parental home to form an independent household. Many young people had started families of their own by their early twenties (Morrow and Richards 1996; Roberts 1995). Within traditional youth transitions two main strands were regarded as of fundamental importance: leaving education to enter the labour market, and leaving what Wallace terms 'the family of origin' (living with parents) to start 'families of destination' (Wallace 1987).

Youth research in the 1980s and 1990s has documented the growth of what have been termed extended and fractured transitions (Coles 1995; Furlong and Cartmel 1997; Jones and Wallace 1992; Morrow and Richards 1996). Extended transitions refer to the longer time period over which young people enter the labour market and/or begin to live independently, and research in this area has tended to focus on problems within educational and labour markets which hinder the first move into secure long-term employment. In particular, studies have focused on the reproduction of inequalities of access to education and the labour market. An abundance of research evidence suggests that patterns of post-16 education or training which were most likely to lead to positive outcomes later in the life course were associated with young people with a middle-class background, and were mediated by educational success and good qualifications at the age of 16 (Banks *et al.* 1992; Furlong 1992; Roberts 1993). There is also evidence of the ways in which training schemes and vocational education have reflected and reproduced a gender-stratified labour market: young women were being socialised into 'caring jobs' or secretarial, catering, selling and personal services; and young men were offered access to a wider range of jobs in industry or trades (Ashton *et al.* 1990; Bates and Riseborough 1993; Coles 1995; Griffin 1985; Skeggs 1990, 1997). Further sub-divisions have also been identified as affecting ethnic minority groups. In Liverpool, for instance, one study found that whilst 50 per cent of white youth were employed by the age of 18–19 and 20 per cent were unemployed, these figures were almost exactly reversed for the city's black youth. This trend could not be accounted for in terms of educational attainment or residential concentration adjacent to collapsed labour markets (Connolly *et al.* 1992). Regional differences were also very marked, especially at the height of the mid-1980s recession. Ashton *et al.* (1988) found that the chances of unemployment amongst young men in Sunderland were one in three compared to one in 33 in St Albans – levels that far outweighed class differences. However, much of the evidence on the growth of extended transitions was based on an examination of educational and labour market experience alone, with little attempt to examine the consequences for families of longer periods of family dependency. This tendency overlooked or relegated the importance of the other two transition strands concerning housing and family relationships.

Research on fractured transitions, however, generally has a wider remit which encompasses the study of youth unemployment and youth homelessness. This area of research recognises that many young people may leave full-time education and training without obtaining employment; may leave the parental home without securing alternative accommodation; and may become isolated from familial or surrogate family and welfare state support. Some studies of vulnerable groups – including chapters in this volume – suggest a complex relationship between employment, domestic and housing transitions (Coles 1997; MacDonald 1997; Biehal and Wade, this volume; Speak, this volume). For instance, care leavers are often required to live independently at the age of 16 or 17 and many become parents in their teens. In these circumstances concern over securing accommodation and stabilising domestic circumstances means that post-16 education and/or employment is less of a pressing priority (Baldwin 1998). By contrast, young people with special educational needs are much more likely to experience extended transitions involving further education and training, despite the fact that they are unlikely to gain employment. Furthermore, most young people in this category will be expected to return to live in the family home despite formal training in independent living (Baldwin *et al.* 1997; Mitchell 1998). For other groups the evidence is less clear cut. There is, for instance, a growing concern about 'status zero' 16- and 17-year-olds, a term coined to identify young people who are not in any form of education, work or training and who have no known independent form of income (Pierce and Hillman 1998; Williamson 1997). Many of these young people also experience homelessness and detachment from families (Hall 1996). The dynamics of how young people reach this status remain unclear, although some research points towards the cumulative effect of numerous, small, and often unplanned chaotic events in young people's lives, some of which are more related to their family circumstances than to a deliberate attempt to shun employment, training or education (Williamson 1997). The complexities of these interactions suggest that social research needs to be careful and more vigilant about the relationship between family and housing factors and education and labour market experiences (Catan 1998).

The growth in both extended and fractured transitions also led youth researchers to separate out at least three different, but related, transition strands: the school-to-work transition; the domestic transition – moving from family of origin to family of destination;

and the housing transition, in which young people move away from the family home eventually to form households of their own (Coles 1995; Jones and Wallace 1992). The conceptual separation of the domestic and housing transitions also highlights questions about the meaning of home and the complexity of the process of leaving home. Jones proposes that the concept of home involves both the physical space of where someone lives, and sets of social and emotional relationships which might include dependency and mutual support (Jones 1995a). Thus, young people following extended transitions in education and training may physically 'leave home' in the sense that they live in accommodation away from their parents, but for many such a move does not preclude a continuation of dependency on and expectation of support from the parents. Indeed, as will be seen later in the chapter, the physical move may be regarded as temporary since the young person might return home during vacations and might move back home on a more permanent basis after course work or training is completed.

Extended transitions and family relationships

Relatively few studies in recent years have specifically focused on the family relationships of young people living at home. Where this has been included as a significant dimension of empirical research, most attention has been focused on the impact of unemployment on family relationships (Allatt and Yeandle 1992; Coffield *et al.* 1986; Hutson and Jenkins 1989; Wallace 1987). For instance, in the mid-1980s Hutson and Jenkins studied 58 families drawn from three areas in South Wales. The main focus of this study was on how families coped when sons and daughters were unemployed. Within the sample of families, conflict between young people and parents was widespread although unemployment *per se* was not found to be the primary cause of such conflict. Many young people were well aware that they continued to live at home on sufferance, and that this was often dependent upon brittle and disputed negotiations about their responsibilities and behaviour. Money, the lack of it, and the use to which it was put, was often at the forefront of family disputes which, given that many of the parents themselves were not in work, is hardly surprising. Paying 'board money' has been noted by a number of studies to be an important symbolic exchange, through which young people negotiate a more adult status *vis-à-vis* their parents (Jones 1995a). Yet changes in entitlement to benefit means that those young people who are unemployed and living at home have only a very restricted means of being able to enter into such negotiation (Smith *et al.* 1998).

Domestic bargaining was also an important issue, although young women were required to do more in terms of housework, in recognition of their continued staying at home. Research by Smith *et al.* drew similar conclusions, and found that parents' willingness to provide a home to adult children became conditional on their observing an informal contract specifying reasonable behaviour (Smith *et al.* 1998). Hutson and Jenkins (1989) also illustrated how young people continuing to live at home whilst unemployed had severe consequences for the welfare of other family members. Not least of these involved overcrowding, with brothers and sisters being denied access to private space as they grew up because of the continued presence of young people living in the family home well into their twenties. Amongst the sample of young unemployed living at home, Hutson and Jenkins found some who had gained brief periods of employment, and some who had left home at some stage only to return later. A young person being in work made a substantial impact on household relationships: the income generated, their ability to pay board, and their being out of the house and away from other family members for significant stretches of the day and week all considerably enhanced family relationships and avoided generational conflict. Similar improvements were also experienced when young people were able to move out. Any return to live in the parental home was often an unwilling one, and was usually a consequence of not being able to continue to afford the cost of living independently. Even in their mid-twenties, some young people were forced by circumstances to return to live at home and their families reluctantly accepted that the family home was still their last refuge.

Outside the context of youth unemployment, Finch and Mason have highlighted the importance of understanding the ways in which relationships within families are negotiated, the assumptions on which such negotiations take place, and the interface between the cultures and practices of family obligation and social policy assumptions about them (Finch 1989; Finch and Mason 1993). Finch and Mason argue that assumptions about the obligations of parents to care for children and young people are deeply embedded in a range of social policies which, increasingly since the 1980s, have attempted to redraw the boundaries about the different, competing or overlapping responsibilities of the family and the welfare state. In their empirical work, they demonstrated that, within a general sample of parents, there is no wide-ranging consensus about the sorts of circumstances in which parents should give support for older children in providing them with somewhere to live, financial support in meeting their everyday needs, or social and emotional support in times of crisis. Jones's detailed exploration of family support for young people leaving home also demonstrated considerable variability in the ability of parents to give in financial, emotional or material terms. In particular, Jones documented two main factors which stand in the way of extended family support. First, some parents are simply not in a position to give: they may be unemployed or on limited incomes, have to think about their commitments to other children, or have financial commitments to more than one family. Second, family obligations are very difficult to negotiate, especially where family tension already exists and where one parent may be a step-parent. Young people are also uncertain and unclear about what they can legitimately expect from their parents, or for how long (Jones 1995a).

THE SOCIAL POLICY CONTEXT OF EXTENDED TRANSITIONS

Many studies have noted the increased incidence of extended transitions, and secondary analysis of the *Survey of English Housing* illustrates the acute nature of this change. Much of the growth in young people living at home occurred in the early 1990s. Within the 20–24 year old age group, in the late 1970s, 52 per cent of men and 31 per cent of women were living in the parental home, a pattern which had changed only slightly by 1991. However, since 1991 there has been a sharp upturn: by 1996/7, 60 per cent of young men and 38 per cent of young women were living with their parents, a proportionate increase of 20 per cent and 19 per cent respectively (Holmans 1996, secondary analysis of SEH). Rugg and Burrows (this volume) have used the SEH to draw out the gender, age, household and tenure characteristics of young people still living with their parents. In summary, the people in this group were more likely to be men, who tended to remain in the parental home until their early to mid-twenties. Young women were much more likely to have left home by this time. Where 16–25 year olds were living with lone parents, it was more probable that they would be living in social housing rather than in owner occupation.

Growth in the incidence of extended transitions is further evidenced by the numbers of young people in post-compulsory education and training. In 1974 nearly two-thirds of 16-year-olds were in employment, but by 1984 the proportion in work had reduced to less than one in five and ten years later had reduced further to one in ten (Roberts 1984, 1993). The collapse of the youth labour market in the 1970s resulted first in a very rapid expansion of youth training, in which more than a quarter of 16- and 17-year-olds participated in the mid-1980s. More recently, post-16 education has been subject to growth, and now includes four-fifths of 16–18-year-olds and a third of young people over the age of 18. Thus the proportion of over-16s who are financially dependent upon their parents for longer has more than doubled in less than a decade.

Explanations for the growth in extended transitions have been found in changes to both the housing market and the youth labour market. In terms of housing, there has been a contraction in the types of property which young people have previously found accessible, and in the ability of young people to afford the rents charged in the private rented sector (Rugg, this volume). Most young people are not a priority group in housing allocations in social housing, and there has been a reduced availability of housing stock suitable for young single people (Anderson, this volume). Clearly, delaying entry into the labour market until their early twenties means that young people before that age do not have access to an income able to finance independent housing. Even when in employment, the income levels of young men are less than the average for all men in manual groups, and those of young women considerably less again. Unless other family members are able to subsidise a young person's attempt to live independently, it is highly unlikely that they will be able to afford to do so until they have obtained secure and well-paid employment, and saved sufficiently to afford the start-up costs of an independent home.

For many commentators, however, the principal factor implicated in the growth of extended transitions has been a series of welfare and benefit reforms that have targeted young people for cuts in support (Coles 1995; Craig 1991; Harris 1989; Jones 1995b; Maclagan 1993; Rugg, this volume). Key amongst these policy changes are the 1986 and 1988 Social Security Acts. The 1986 Act, implemented in 1988, replaced the old Supplementary Benefit with Income Support but removed entitlement for Income Support from 16- and 17-year-olds. A different rate was also set for claimants under the age of 25. These changes have been continued under the Job Seekers Allowance introduced in 1996. Prior to 1988, Supplementary Benefit was based upon a distinction between householders and non-householders in calculating entitlement. The new assessments explicitly assume that the financial responsibilities and needs of young people who are unemployed and under the age of 25 differ from those of older age groups: assessment is based on age alone rather than needs or financial obligations. The withdrawal of benefit entitlement from 16- and 17-year-olds was done explicitly in tandem with the introduction of a 'youth training guarantee': everyone in that age group who was not in full-time education was guaranteed a place on youth training. Some commentators have argued that the withdrawal of benefit was also specifically designed as both a work incentive and as a means of discouraging young people from leaving the parental home (Jones 1991; Roll 1990).

Research undertaken since the implementation of the Act has consistently shown both that the guarantee is not being met, and that a significant number of young people are estranged from their parents and cannot reasonably be expected to look to them for financial support (Chatrik 1996; Craig 1991; Killeen 1992; Maclagan 1993). Some attempt to remedy this trend was made in 1988 with the introduction of the Youth Training Bridging Allowance and Severe Hardship Payment (SHP) which was intended to address the needs of what were anticipated as being a small number of deserving cases. Yet between 1989 and 1992, applications for SHP increased by 300 per cent, and in 1992 nearly two-thirds of applications were for repeat and continuous claims (Maclagan 1993). However, application for SHP involves young people having to provide incontrovertible evidence that they are registered with the careers service as looking for work or a training place, and that they are irretrievably estranged from their parents. As a consequence, payments are by no means easy to secure (Castles 1997; McManus 1998). These benefit changes have led to a climate in which leaving the parental home can be viewed as an extremely precarious business, with state benefits unlikely to provide much assistance in helping young people to settle in secure accommodation away from the family home.

Policy changes in education, and particularly higher education, have also brought about longer periods of family dependency. For many students, especially in England and Wales, going to college or university involves the first move away from the parental home. Yet the gradual erosion of the maintenance grant, the introduction of student loans to meet the shortfall and, since 1997, tuition fees for undergraduates, means that young people who benefit from higher education do so at both considerable expense to their families and the accumulation of debt to themselves. It is estimated that the average debt accumulation by undergraduates is now of the order of £10,000 (*Times Educational Supplement* 14.8.98). Whilst having a degree may qualify young people to enter a more lucrative – if sometimes insecure and precarious – graduate labour market, increasingly students embark upon such employment careers with responsibility to pay off debts and loans. The full impact of these trends may not be felt for some years, but it seems likely that for some young graduates returning to live in the parental home will, at least in the short term, be the only affordable option.

Thus broad shifts in policy, including labour market and benefit and education changes, are all pushing in the same direction: towards further extending youth transitions and requiring longer periods of dependency upon the family. It is important to note that during the same period in which the family dependency of young people increased both in length and volume, family structures themselves have become more brittle. Although the overwhelming majority of children still live with two parents, many family structures change during the time children grow up. It is therefore important to map the dynamics of family change onto static pictures of the distribution of family types. Since the 1960s there has been more than a doubling of the number of lone parent families, a four-fold increase in the number of divorces and a threefold growth of remarriages. If these dynamics are taken into account, by the time they reach the age of 16 only around half of young people will still be living with both their married biological parents (Keirnan and Wicks 1990). The implications of this trend in terms of family dependency remain unclear, although research by Jones indicates that family support was least likely to be forthcoming where parents were unemployed or had undergone separation or divorce (Jones 1995a).

YOUNG PEOPLE LIVING IN THE PARENTAL HOME

Although it is clear that young people are living in the parental home for longer, statistics illustrating the growing trend in favour of living at home often fail to represent the complexity of young people's individual housing histories. Policy needs to acknowledge that young people living at home are not a homogeneous group. As has been indicated, Jones makes clear that early housing careers are not linear, and a proportion of 16–25 year olds living with their parents will be returners. Citing figures from the National Child Development Study, Jones notes that at the age of 23 30 per cent of men and 38 per cent of women living in the parental home had previously lived independently (Jones 1995b: 63). Thus any assessment of the nature and experience of young people living with their parents has to take 'non-leavers' and 'returners' into account. Analysis of young people living in the countryside completed by Ford *et al.* (1997) indicates that further refinement can be given to this classification to distinguish between 'committed stayers', 'committed leavers', 'reluctant stayers' and 'reluctant leavers'. This chapter recognises two further sub-groups: young people living at home who have not yet made any housing decisions; and students who live part of the year away at college or university and part of the year in the parental home. Six different groups should therefore be distinguished:

- 'pre-decision' stayers;
- willing stayers;
- reluctant stayers;
- reluctant returners;
- willing returners; and
- students studying away from home.

These classifications take into account both the housing histories of young people and their expectations and preferences. The categories are not tightly bounded: as much of the chapter will show, there is considerable shading and overlap between sub-groups, and young people may shift from one group to another a number of times in the course of staying with their parents. For these reasons, estimates cannot be given of numbers and proportions of young people in each group. However, the groupings do offer a useful way of exploring the different populations of young people living in the parental home.

'Pre-decision' stayers

In their 1994 analysis of the effects of benefit on housing decisions, Kemp *et al.* completed exploratory interviews with a small number of young people living with their parents. The study made a distinction between 'voluntary' and 'involuntary' stayers within the parental home, but in the former category recognised that some of the young people who were interviewed clearly had not thought at all about their housing situation. When asked why they never thought of leaving, some found it difficult to frame an answer. The report gave the example of one young man who at the age of 25 had not thought about his housing situation at all: he said 'I don't know, I just haven't. I suppose I'm happy.' The report concluded that in some cases young people did not question their continuing to live in the parental home, largely because they had no reason to do so. For this reason, the group can be judged as neither committed nor reluctant stayers. Ongoing research by Jones and Rugg amongst young people in North Yorkshire (Jones, this volume) is revealing similar attitudes amongst some of the interviewees still living at home: little thought had been given to the notion of leaving simply because the issue had never arisen. Studies of leaving home confirm that, for the most part, young people need a reason to move out of the parental home (Jones 1995b). The young people in the Kemp *et al.* (1994) study who had not thought about their housing anticipated that they would probably only do so when they wanted to move in with a partner.

Very little is known about young adults who are living in the parental home and who have yet to make any housing decisions, and research has yet to be completed which estimates the size of this sub-group within the population still living with their parents. Some issues do attach to this group. For example, it is important to understand the extent to which these young people understand their possible housing options or have realistic housing expectations. In the early 1990s, a small-scale survey of the housing expectations of schoolchildren in four schools in Kendal, Reading, Sheffield and Maltby indicated great variation in the anticipated costs of accommodation, with estimates ranging from £5 to £200 a week (Darke *et al.* 1993: 22). An increased value has been attached to the need for pre-school leavers to receive education on housing matters. In 1985 the then Department of the Environment issued a Code of Guidance on the homelessness legislation, which noted that local education authorities should work with housing authorities to ensure that housing and homelessness projects were included in the curriculum. These projects would give young people 'a realistic idea of the implications of leaving home and living independently, and of the potential pitfalls' (quoted in Oxley 1993: 4). Since that time, a number of voluntary sector housing agencies have recognised the need for school projects on housing issues as a means of preventing homelessness. For example Shelter's Network Project, which looked at local strategies for tackling housing need amongst young people, issued a teachers' guide on housing for distribution to secondary schools (Morton 1998), whilst Ford *et al.* (1997) noted school-based work by rural housing agencies.

Willing stayers

Closely connected to the 'pre-decision' stayers are the young people who have actively chosen to continue living at home. Researchers have pointed out that it is very difficult to disentangle positive attitudes towards living at home from the pragmatic realisation that other alternatives are financially untenable (Burton *et al.* 1989a). Indeed, living at home appears not only a relatively cheap option compared with other housing possibilities but in some cases an option with absolutely minimal financial commitment. Although most young people are asked by their parents for board money, the sums asked for generally reflect a symbolic payment rather than a figure that represents the real cost of their living at home (Wallace 1987). However, it is unreasonable to expect that young people's willingness to stay at home is influenced entirely by economic motivations. The young 'voluntary stayers' in the Kemp *et al.* (1994) study generally valued living at home and being close to their family. A large-scale study of shared accommodation by Green and Holroyd (1992) came to similar conclusions. Although 55 per cent of its sample of under-thirties gave being unable to afford an alternative as one reason for staying with their parents, 77 per cent agreed strongly that they liked being in the parental home.

Within the sub-groupings of young people living with their parents, it is difficult to judge the willing stayers as anything but unproblematic, at least for the young people themselves. The willingness to stay can be assumed to some degree to rest on good relationships with other family members, and if in work this group is likely to have a reasonable level of disposable income. However, these are assumed characterisations rather than conclusions drawn from extensive research. The apparently settled nature of this group does not preclude the need for study, especially given a policy imperative to recreate all under-25s as contented homestayers. It would be possible to continue forcing young people to continue to live in or return to the parental home by reducing access to assistance with independent housing costs, or further educating pre-school leavers on the limited nature of their housing choices; but a willingness to remain at home often rests on quite complex family dynamics that would be impossible for policy makers to replicate through regulation.

Reluctant stayers

A number of young people living in the parental home can be judged as being reluctant or involuntary stayers: they remain at home because they cannot find alternative accommodation. Much of this volume has explored the obstacles to entering the main tenures, and it is unnecessary to repeat this material here. Quantifying the number of reluctant stayers is difficult. To some degree, this group becomes part of a separate housing debate that attempts to assess the number of what has been termed 'hidden homeless' people: individuals in housing need, but whose housing situation has not yet become so desperate that they have to make recourse to sleeping in hostels or on the street (Watson and Austerberry 1986). Much of the difficulty with quantification rests with definition and degree. The housing need of young people will range on a continuum of acuteness: at one extreme, for example, their parents may have told them to leave, and given them a non-negotiable time-scale in which to do so; at the other extreme, the young person may simply be unhappy with their housing situation but not be under any pressure to find somewhere else to live.

Although there is a good understanding of the structural forces that compel young people to remain in the parental home, and extensive research has been completed on the 'crisis' points that may provoke a sometimes hasty move out, little is known about the young people who are unhappy with living at home, despite so doing. It may be that the reluctance rests in the simple desire for independence, which tends not to formulate itself into a lifecourse 'event' that would provoke a move – such as taking up a job or living with a partner. The desire to become independent is, rather, a feeling that may fluctuate over time but will at some juncture reach the stage at which the young person will decide that it is no longer appropriate for them to continue living with their parents: a willing stayer then becomes an unwilling stayer. Although work in this area has not been completed, it is important that this shift is explored to understand which types of young people and what circumstances provoke earlier or later desire for living independently.

In addition, it is probable that a proportion of the reluctant stayers have previously made some attempts to leave, and further research needs to be completed about the nature of these failed attempts. Kemp and Rugg's study of young people on Housing Benefit found that many had problems securing accommodation, but the biggest difficulties were faced by young people attempting to move out of the parental home (Kemp and Rugg 1998). Most of these young people looked for accommodation over a period of months. The assumption remains that these attempts to move out fail because of structural factors in different housing markets. It must also be the case that some young people who are looking for the first time are simply not experienced enough to know which possible alternatives to explore. For example, Kemp *et al.* (1994) found one case in their small sample, of a young woman whose ignorance of benefit entitlements meant that she continued to live with her parents – in very overcrowded circumstances – because she did not realise that Housing Benefit would supplement her low income and help her afford a private rent. She had spent months fruitlessly looking for a rent her low wage could cover. The lack of research in this area also means that very limited information is available on what sort of housing young people first want to move into, and how far a direct shift from the parental home affects their choice – perhaps by limiting what might otherwise be considered reasonable options. For example, the Kemp and Rugg (1998) report indicated that young people favoured the notion of going directly into shared accommodation since they felt they would otherwise be lonely, having been used to living with their parents and siblings.

Reluctant returners

A sub-group closely associated with the unwilling stayers is the reluctant returners. These are young people who have moved out of the parental home for a range of reasons, but have had to return – often because of a failure to sustain an independent tenancy. Jones (1995b) notes a general shift in favour of a greater number of young people returning home, and notes research which suggests a possible explanation in the decreased frequency of young people leaving to get married. Using data from the National Child Development Study, Jones found a higher frequency of returns home where the young person had left to take up a job (52 per cent return) or to study (48 per cent return), compared with those leaving to set up home with a partner (11 per cent return) (Jones 1995b: 64). As with those young people willingly remaining in the parental home, the degree to which a young person may make a willing or unwilling return after an experience of independent living becomes a difficult judgement to make. However, it is possible to note the incidence of reasons for returning that are due to factors 'over which the young person may have no control. For example, 'financial reasons' are cited as a reason for returning by 34 per cent of young people who had initially left home because of family problems, and given as the cause of return by 50 per cent of the young people who had left because they wanted to live independently. The problems under the category of 'financial' reasons are likely to be wide ranging. For example, Ford et al.'s 1997 study reported two young men who had managed to move into rented accommodation: they could meet the rental costs, but were not able to afford to furnish their place, or meet amenity bills and so reluctantly had to return home (Ford et al. 1997). Jones notes that of the young people leaving to take up a particular job, 48 per cent returned because the job finished; 14 per cent returned because they had become unemployed; and 11 per cent returned for financial reasons (Jones 1995b: 67).

It is clear that, in Jones's study, a proportion of reluctant returners have been able to use the parental home as a safety net, thus confirming some policy makers' contentions that in times of difficulty young people can always go home (Rugg, this volume). However, questions remain about this population of returners, and the impact of their experience of independent living on the resumption of a stay in the parental home and subsequent willingness to leave. Each young person will be more or less able to cope with shifts in and out of independence, but it may be reasonable to assume that as the young person becomes older, or the periods of independence more protracted, then a return to the parental home becomes less appropriate. In economic terms, the young person may have made a financial commitment to property which will be lost as a consequence of a return to the parental home, perhaps including entry costs to owner occupation and costs of furnishing and decoration. In less tangible terms, the young person's experience of independent living means that it is more difficult for them to resume the role of a dependant within their parents' household, with the concomitant implicit return to childhood. Kemp and Rugg's study of young people on Housing Benefit noted the experience of a 23-year-old man, who had returned to live with his mother whilst he was between private tenancies. When they argued, she still sent him to his room. Although he laughed about the experience, he did not stay much longer than two weeks (Kemp and Rugg 1998).

Willing returners

By contrast, some young people willingly return to the parental home: the option remains less a safety net and more a haven from difficult experiences with independent living. Jones recognises at least two types of willing returner, which include those whose leaving was always intended to be temporary (perhaps because of short-term contract work away from home), and those whose 'problematic' reasons for leaving had become resolved. Thus, of the young people who had left because of difficulties with their family, 41 per cent later returned because their family wanted them to come back (Jones 1995b: 67). Mention is also made of loneliness as a reason for returning, further indicating that the family home carries emotional values which young people obviously take into account when deciding where to live. Even where family relationships may be tense, the home could constitute a location in which young people maintain social networks which they do not want to lose.

In a more general sense, research needs to be completed of the contrasting housing histories of the willing and reluctant returners before categorical statements can be made about the impact of a spell of independent living on young people's periods of stay in the parental home. It is uncertain what is 'learned' from the experience of living away: for example, after a bad independent housing

experience in their early twenties, some young people might not con-
template moving away again for some years; or alternatively a 'taste'
for independence might mean that reluctant returners move out
again after only a few months.

Students studying away from home

A sixth sub-group of young people living in the parental home are
students who spend part of their year studying away from home.
As Rhodes (this volume) demonstrates, full-time students are a
growing proportion of young people. During their time of study
this group does not readily fit into any of the other five classifications, although at the time of graduation students might judge themselves to be in any one of the categories. Ongoing research by Jones
and Rugg, looking at the housing and employment decisions of
young people living in rural North Yorkshire (Jones, this volume),
found that many young people's movement into higher education
was a career rather than a housing decision and at that time of
interview (all young people in the sample were interviewed at the
age of 21) they had yet to consider any long-term housing options.
When asked if they had left the parental home, some students did
not think they had, even though they may have spent three or
more terms in the private rented sector: for them, consistent returns
to the parental home remained more significant.

A number of questions have yet to be answered about the way in
which the experience of being a student affects young people's early
housing histories. More than any other group, students experience a
largely supported move to independent living in being provided, for
at least the first year of their course, with accommodation in halls of
residence or similar housing that is largely supervised. Even in their
'year out' of halls, Rhodes (this volume) indicates the degree to
which students have advantages over their non-student peers with
respect to institutional support. The conventions of being a student
mean that for some of the year they have access to the parental home
that, for the most part, does not have to be negotiated: in complying
with their children going into higher education, parents tacitly
agreed to continue to house their children for three or more years.
In these respects, it may be concluded that, in housing terms, full-
time students are one of the least vulnerable groups of young
people. The housing situation of students at the point of graduation
is another matter, and research is only now being completed on

housing careers in the months following graduation, within the context of the new fees and grants structures (Rosser 1997). It may be assumed that there will commonly be a more or less willing return to the parental home, especially given the high level of debt most students find themselves in on the completion of their courses. Whether this debt in itself provokes an extended stay in the parental home is too early to tell, given the relatively recent time period in which maintenance grants have been reduced.

Thus, it is clear that generalisations cannot be made about young people living in the parental home and indeed, despite their growing numbers, they have remained a largely under-researched population. For young people, living with their parents will carry some consequences on their early employment experiences and their household formation decisions, but limitations of space preclude discussion of these areas. This next section, rather, speculates on the consequences of a heavy reliance on the parental home to house young people.

HOUSING YOUNG PEOPLE IN THE PARENTAL HOME: A POLICY AGENDA

Young people continuing to live at home has rarely been seen as a problem to be addressed by social policy. Indeed continuing to live at home, with resultant longer family dependency, closer parental supervision and intensive parental support for young people, has more often been seen as a solution to many youth policy problems rather than creating issues which policy makers ought to address. In the case of younger children and families, extensive legislation seeks to define when it is the responsibility of the state to intervene, for what reasons, and in what way to regulate and 'normalise' family relationships (Department of Health 1991). Yet, as Finch and Mason rightly point out, there is some contradiction in family policy: on the one hand family responsibility is considered part of family life, but on the other hand it is accepted that the state has a role in enforcing such responsibilities, so implying that these may not be universally regarded as 'natural' (Finch and Mason 1993). Many parents have accepted their teenage and adult children living at home, although at significant cost to themselves and other family members. It is clear that a number of social policy and housing policy issues relating to extended stays in the parental home need to be addressed. The limited number of empirical studies of young people continuing to live at home suggests the need for a research agenda. In particular, policy making requires more accurate intelligence on the size of the different groups living with their parents, the interplay of reasons why young people may remain in the parental home, the barriers they face in contemplating living away from home, and the life course consequences – for them and other family members – of being forced to continue to live at home reluctantly. In addition, five main housing issues may be recognised as being central to any new research on housing and young people.

First, it is clear that many of those continuing to live at home are an important, though rarely recognised, sub-group of the 'hidden homeless'. They are often living in overcrowded accommodation, and in domestic relationships which are stressful for everyone concerned. Where such relationships break down, then young people will leave in an often unplanned way, and with few material, emotional or financial supports to protect them against the likelihood of homelessness (Jones 1995b). A failure to address the needs of the hidden homeless, therefore, may be one of the reasons why homelessness proves to be such an intractable problem, despite initiatives to develop provision for more obvious homeless groups living in hostels or on the streets. Policy makers need to pay attention to issues of prevention as well as cure when addressing the continued problem of homelessness.

Second, many young people continuing to live at home are unemployed: indeed a number of studies have indicated that unemployment increases the likelihood of staying with parents. Furthermore, amongst the young unemployed living at home, there is also some noted spatial concentrations of unemployment. On social housing estates, for instance, not only are there concentrations of the young unemployed, but over half the young people live in households in which there is no adult in employment (Power and Tunstall 1995; Coles *et al.* 1998). The lack of alternative accommodation means that young people are spatially and domestically trapped in communities adjacent to collapsed labour markets and not in a position to seek employment in other areas where there may be work. These young people comprise an important sub-group of all those experiencing the 'no-home-no-job' cycle. Research being undertaken in rural Scotland suggests that this spatial entrapment of young people is not confined to social housing estates in urban areas, but is an important feature of rural communities (Furlong and Cartmel, forthcoming). The growth of foyers is one development attempting to address how to break the 'no-home-no-job' cycle (Anderson and Quilgars 1995), yet it is unlikely that these alone will provide an appropriate answer to the needs of the group currently living at home.

Third, this chapter has drawn attention to the potential and real adverse family outcomes of continuing to house young adults in the family home. These consequences can take various forms, and can include financial hardship for the family. Leaving home does not necessarily release housing space in the accommodation young people leave. Insecurities in the youth labour and housing markets mean that families may maintain empty rooms or larger-than-necessary family homes in order to keep a place for young people who are undergoing temporary higher education or training. To be able to meet a responsibility to house an adult child, parents have to maintain reserved space in the family household: essentially they have to manage a 'void', which carries some financial cost. If the parents are living in owner occupation they will have to carry the mortgage and rating costs of a home that would probably be in excess of their needs. For parents in social housing, the family would be considered 'over accommodated', and in instances where pressure for family housing is high, lone parents in particular may be asked to accept a transfer to a smaller dwelling. In the limited number of instances of parents living in the private rented sector, if they were in receipt of Housing Benefit, their entitlement would not cover the extra rental cost of the 'spare' room.

Fourth, this chapter has pointed to the ways in which continuing to live at home creates conflict within the family, not only between young people and their parents but also with other family members. Where young people living at home are doing so in high unemployment areas they are also likely to be living in families with a larger than average family size, and in overcrowded accommodation (Coles *et al.* 1998). Hutson and Jenkins (1989) commented on the ways in which this created competition within the household for private living space, and the ways in which younger children were denied access to their own rooms which remained allocated to older teenagers and young people in their twenties who continued to live at home. For both these groups, this competition for space at home, and the inability to afford to take part in in-door leisure facilities, forces them out onto the streets. One of the major complaints people make of young people living in social housing estates is of large congregations of young people 'hanging around' (Coles *et al.* 1998). This, and police acting on the complaints they received, has also be shown to be one of the main causes of social disturbance (Power and Tunstall 1997). Yet policy on disorder on social housing estates seems more inclined to address the symptoms – including children and young people out on the streets – rather than the causes, which are overcrowded homes and no affordable alternative space.

A fifth issue relates to the difficulties young people face in all sectors of the housing market: their inability to compete with others, to afford to sustain the costs of independent housing and their lack of preparation for independent living. If, as many of the chapters in this book have illustrated, young people have only a precarious and costly foothold in forms of transitional housing, it must be expected that more and more young people will be forced back into the parental home as a last resort. Increasingly young people will have no alternative but to remain living at home until such time as they think they can afford to move straight into private housing. Yet little attention is given to preparing them for such a move or managing the cost of so doing. At least in part as a result of this lack of preparation there have been increasing numbers of people unable to keep up with their mortgages: repossessions of properties by building societies are estimated to be over a thousand households per week (Ford *et al.* 1995b), with households headed by a young person under the age of 30 being amongst those most at risk of indebtedness (Burrows 1998).

CONCLUSIONS

Much of the burgeoning literature on young transitions has concentrated upon the impact of labour market changes, youth training and trends in post-compulsory education. This literature has helped document both the decline in traditional transitions and the incidence of fractured transitions, resulting in disaffection from education, training and employment, long-term youth unemployment, youth homelessness and the breakdown of family support and social care. Research relating to these complex processes have also added to an understanding of the growth of longer periods of family dependency. The 1990s in particular have seen an increase in the incidence of extended transitions, with young people remaining in the parental home for longer, awaiting appropriate housing and employment opportunities to enable them to achieve independent living.

This chapter has highlighted the policy context in which the growth in extended transitions has occurred. Many of the policies to which this chapter has referred are based on an assumption that longer periods of family dependency are both an inevitable and desirable outcome of social and economic change. This chapter questions such assumptions and draws attention to the variety of circumstances in which young people continue to live at home. Some young people and their families are content with such arrangements. But there are other circumstances which suggest that continuing to live at home disguises youth homelessness, a widespread existence of the 'no-home-no-job' syndrome, spatial concentrations of poverty, community breakdown, and poor preparation for later housing careers. Far from being a social policy solution to a number of youth policy issues, young people living at home for longer may constitute both the evidence for and cause of problems relating to young people's movement in the housing market. This conclusion points to the urgent need to create a new policy agenda addressing the needs of young people in the housing market: this chapter and this book have begun to define such an agenda.

References

Ainley, P. (1991) *Young People Leaving Home*, London: Cassell.

Allatt, P. and Yeandle, S. (1992) *Youth Unemployment and the Family: Voices of Disordered Times*, London: Routledge.

Allen, T. (1994) *Which University 1995*, Cambridge: Hobsons.

Anderson, I. (1994) *Access to Housing for Low Income Single People*, York: Centre for Housing Policy, University of York.

—— (1997) 'Housing for young people', *Housing Review*, 46, 4, July–August, pp. 76–7.

Anderson, I. and Douglas, A. (1998) *The Development of Foyers in Scotland*, Edinburgh: Scottish Homes.

Anderson, I. and Morgan, J. (1997) *Social Housing for Single People: a Study of Local Policy and Practice*, Stirling: Housing Policy and Practice Unit, University of Stirling.

Anderson, I. and Quilgars, D. (1995) *Foyers for Young People: Evaluation of a Pilot Initiative*, York: Centre for Housing Policy, University of York.

Anderson, I., Kemp, P. A. and Quilgars, D. (1993) *Single Homeless People*, London: HMSO.

Ashton, D. (1989) 'Youth and labour markets', in Gallie, D. (ed.) *Employment in Britain*, Oxford: Basil Blackwell.

Ashton, D. N., Maguire, M. and Spilsbury, M. (1988) 'Local labour markets and their impact on the life-chances of youths', in Coles, B. (ed.) *Young Careers: Youth Unemployment and the New Vocationalism*, Buckingham: Open University Press.

—— (1990) *Restructuring the Labour Market: the Implications for Youth*, London: Macmillan.

Balchin, P. (1995) *Housing Policy: an Introduction* (3rd edition), London: Routledge.

Baldwin, D. (1998) 'Growing up in and out of care: an ethnographic approach to young people's transitions to adulthood', Unpublished Ph.D. thesis, University of York.

Baldwin, D., Coles, B. and Mitchell, W. (1997) 'The formation of an underclass or disparate processes of social exclusion? Evidence from two groupings of "vulnerable youth"', in MacDonald, R. (ed.) *Youth, the Underclass and Social Exclusion*, London: Routledge.

Banks, M., Bates, I., Breakwell, G., Bynner, J., Emler, N., Jamieson, L. and Roberts, K. (1992) *Careers and Identities*, Buckingham: Open University Press.

Barclay, P. M. (1985) *Fourth Report of the Social Security Advisory Committee*, London: HMSO.

Bates, I. and Riseborough, G. (eds) (1993) *Youth and Inequality*, Buckingham: Open University Press.

Beck, U. (1992) *The Risk Society: Towards a New Modernity*, London: Sage.

Berghman, J. (1995) 'Social exclusion in Europe: policy context and analytical framework', in Room, G. (ed.) *Beyond the Threshold*, Bristol: The Policy Press.

Bevan, M. and Sanderling, L. (1996) *Private Renting in Rural Areas*, York: Centre for Housing Policy, University of York.

Bevan, M., Kemp, P. A. and Rhodes, D. (1995) *Private Landlords and Housing Benefit*, York: Centre for Housing Policy, University of York.

Biehal, N., Clayden, J., Stein, M. and Wade, J. (1992) *Prepared for Living?*, London: National Children's Bureau.

—— (1995) *Moving On: Young People and Leaving Care Schemes*, London: HMSO.

Bovaird, A., Harloe, M. and Whitehead, C. M. E. (1985) 'Private rented housing: its current role', *Journal of Social Policy*, 14, 1, pp. 1–23.

Bramley, G. and Smart, D. (1995) *Rural Incomes and Housing Affordability*, London: Rural Development Commission.

Britain, A. and Yanetta, A. (1997) *Housing Allocations in Scotland – a Practice Note*, Coventry: Chartered Institute of Housing.

British Market Research Bureau (BMRB) (1995) *On the Move*, London: BMRB.

Broad, B. (1994) *Leaving Care in the 1990s*, Westerham: Royal Philanthropic Society.

—— (1998) *Young People Leaving Care*, London: Jessica Kingsley.

Brody, S. (1996) *The Housing Act and Young People – New Guidance*, London: CHAR, National Homeless Alliance.

Brown, T. (1992) 'Inadequate homes for students', *Housing Review*, 41, 6, pp. 100–1.

Burghes, L. and Brown M. (1995) *Single Lone Mothers: Problems, Prospects and Policies*, London: Family Policy Studies Centre.

Burghes, L., Clarke, L. and Cronin, N. (1997) *Fathers and Fatherhood in Britain*, London: Family Policy Studies Centre.

Burrows, R. (1998) 'Mortgage indebtedness in England: an "epidemiology"', *Housing Studies*, 13, 1, pp. 5–22.

Burrows, R., Ford, J., Quilgars, D. and Pleace, N. (1998) 'A place in the country? The housing circumstances of young people in rural England', *Journal of Youth Studies*, 1, 2, pp. 177–94.

Burton, P., Forrest, R. and Stewart, M. (1989a) *Growing up and Leaving Home*, Dublin: The European Foundation for the Improvement of Living and Working Conditions.

—— (1989b) *Urban Environment, Accommodation, Social Cohesion: The Implications for Young People*, Bristol: SAUS, University of Bristol. (PC)

Button, E. (1992) *Rural Housing for Youth*, London: Centrepoint.

Callender, C. and Kempson, E. (1996) *Student Finances: Income, Expenditure and Take-up of Student Loans*, London: Policy Studies Institute.

Campbell, M., Foy, S. and Walton, F. (1996) *Rural Issues in Yorkshire and Humberside*, Leeds: Policy Research Institute.

Carlen, P. (1996) *Jigsaw: A Political Criminology of Youth Homelessness*, Buckingham: Open University Press.

Castles, J. (1997) '16 and 17-year olds: do the existing government policies surrounding employment, training, benefits and housing needs meet the needs of those claiming severe hardship?', MA thesis, Department of Social Policy and Social Work, University of York.

Catan, L. (1998) Review of Brynner, J., Chisholm, L. and Furlong, A., *Youth, Citizenship and Social Change in a European Context*, in *Journal of Youth Studies*, 1, 3, pp. 349–51.

Chatrik, B. (1996) 'Severe hardship claims reach an all-time high', *Working Brief*, 73, pp. 14–15.

Chugg, A. (1998) 'No Entry', unpublished report for the National Federation of Rent Deposit Schemes.

Clark, E. (1989) *Young Single Mothers Today: A Qualitative Study of Housing and Support Needs*, London: National Council For One Parent Families.

Clark, E. and Coleman, J. (1991) *Growing Up Fast. Adult Outcomes of Teenage Motherhood*, London: St. Michael's Fellowship.

Clayden, J. and Stein, M. (1996) 'Self care skills and becoming adult', in Jackson, S. and Kilroe, S. (eds) *Looking After Children: Good Parenting, Good Outcomes*, London: HMSO.

Cloke, P. Milbourne, P. and Thomas, C. (1994) *Lifestyles in Rural England*, Salisbury: Rural Development Commission.

Cloke, P., Goodwin, M., Milbourne, P. and Thomas, C. (1995) 'Deprivation, poverty and marginalization in rural lifestyles in England and Wales', *Journal of Rural Studies*, 11, 4, pp. 351–65.

Coffield, F., Borrill, C. and Marshall, S. (1986) 'Shit jobs, govvy schemes or on the dole: occupational choice for young adults in the North East of England', in Beloff, H. (ed.) *Getting into Life*, London: Methuen.

Coles, B. (1995) *Youth and Social Policy: Youth Citizenship and Young Careers*, London: UCL Press.

—— (1997) 'Vulnerable youth and processes of social exclusion: a theoretical framework, a review of recent research and suggestions for future research agendas', in Brynner, J., Chisholm, L. and Furlong, A. (eds) *Youth, Citizenship and Social Change in a European Context*, Aldershot: Ashgate.

Coles, B., England, J. and Rugg, J. (1998) *Working with Young People on Estates: the Role of Housing Professionals in Multi-agency Work*, Coventry: Chartered Institute of Housing/Joseph Rowntree Foundation.

Committee on Higher Education (1963) *Higher Education*, London: HMSO.

Community Partners (1998) *Skills for Life: A Good Practice Guide to Training Homeless People for Resettlement and Employment*, London: Crisis.

Connolly, M., Roberts, K., Ben-Tovim, G. and Torkington, P. (1992) *Black Youth in Liverpool*, Culemborg, Italy: Giordano Bruno.

Corbett, G. (1998) *The Children (Scotland) Act and Homelessness: the First Six Months*, Edinburgh: Shelter (Scotland).

Cordon, A. and Craig, G. (1991) *Perceptions of Family Credit*, London: HMSO.

Craig, G. (1991) *Fit for Nothing? Young People, Benefits and Youth Training*, London: The Children's Society.

—— (1993) 'Classification and control: the role of the social fund', in Howells, G., Crow, I. and Moroney, M. (eds) *Aspects of Credit and Debt*, London: Sweet and Maxwell.

Craig, T., Hodson, S., Woodward, S. and Richardson, S. (1996) *Off to a Bad Start*, London: The Mental Health Foundation.

CRASH (1996) *Winter Shelters Provided in London*, London: CRASH.

Crook, A. D. H. and Kemp, P. A. (1996) *Private Landlords in England*, London: HMSO.

Crook, A. D. H., Hughes, J. and Kemp, P. A. (1995) *The Supply of Privately Rented Homes: Today and Tomorrow*, York: Joseph Rowntree Foundation.

Currie, H. and Murie, A. (eds) (1996) *Housing in Scotland*, Coventry: Chartered Institute of Housing.

Cutts, R. (1997) 'Priced out of a home: the real cost of the single room rent', unpublished report for the Exeter Homeless Action Group.

Dant, T. and Deacon, A. (1989) *Hostels to Homes? The Rehousing of Single Homeless People*, Aldershot: Avebury.

Darke, J., Conway, J., and Holman, C. with Buckley, K. (1993) *Homes for Our Children*, London: National Housing Forum.

DaVanzo, J. and Goldscheider, F. K. (1990) 'Coming home again: returns to the parental home of young adults', *Population Studies*, 44, pp. 241–55.

Deloitte and Touce Management Advisory Service (1997) *Social Housing, Social Investment*, London: National Housing Federation.

Department of Education and Science (DES) (1988) *Top-up Loans for Students*, London: HMSO.

Department of the Environment (1994) *Access to Local Authority and Housing Association Tenancies, Consultation Paper*, London: HMSO.

Department of the Environment and Ministry of Agriculture, Food and Fisheries (1995) *Rural England: A Nation Committed to a Living Countryside*, London: HMSO.

Department for the Environment, Regions and Transport, Welsh Office and Scottish Office (1997) *Design of the New Deal for 18–24-year olds*, London: Department for the Environment, Regions and Transport, Welsh Office and Scottish Office.

Department of Health (1991) *The Children Act 1989, Guidance and Regulations. Volume 4: Residential Care*, London: HMSO.

—— (1997) *Children Looked After by Local Authorities, Year Ending 31 March 1996*, London: HMSO.

Doling, J., Ford, J. and Stafford, B. (1989) *The Property Owing Democracy*, Aldershot: Avebury.

Dupuis, A. and Thorns, D. (1998) 'Home, home ownership and the search for ontological security', *Sociological Review*, 46, 1, pp. 24–47.

England, J. (forthcoming) *Capital Youth Link: An Evaluation*, London: Capital Housing Project.

Evans, A. (1996) *We Don't Choose to Be Homeless – The Findings of the Inquiry into Preventing Youth Homelessness*, London: CHAR.

Evans, R., Smith, N., Bryson, C. and Austin, N. (1994) *The Code of Guidance on Homelessness in Scotland. Local Authority Policies and Practice*, Edinburgh: Scottish Office Central Research Unit.

Finch, J. (1989) *Family Obligations and Social Change*, Oxford: Polity Press.

Finch, J. and Mason, J. (1993) *Negotiating Family Responsibility*, London: Routledge.

Finer (1974) *The Report of the Committee on One-Parent Families Vol. 1*, London: HMSO.

First Key (1987) *A Study of Black Young People Leaving Care*, Leeds: First Key.

—— (1992) *A Survey of Local Authority Provisions for Young People Leaving Care*, Leeds: First Key.

Ford, J. (1993) 'Mortgage possession', *Housing Studies*, 8, 4, pp. 227–40.

—— (1997) 'As safe as houses?', in Goodwin, J. and Grant, C. (eds) *Built to Last? Reflections on British Housing Policy*, London: Shelter.

Ford, J. and Burrows, R. (1998) 'Attitudes to Owner Occupation and the Labour Market', Discussion Paper, Centre for Housing Policy, University of York.

Ford, J. and Wilcox, S. (1992) *Evaluating the Initiatives: Mortgage Arrears and Possessions*, York: Joseph Rowntree Foundation.

Ford, J., Kempson, E. and England, J. (1995a) *Into Work? The Impact of Housing Costs and Benefits on People's Decision to Work*, York: Joseph Rowntree Foundation.

Ford, J., Kempson, E. and Wilson, M. (1995b) *Mortgage Arrears and Possessions: the Perspective from Lenders, Borrowers and the Courts*, London: HMSO.

Ford, J., Burrows, R., Quilgars, D. and Pleace, N. (1997) *Young People and Housing*, Salisbury: Rural Development Commission.

Forrest, R. and Murie, A. (1983) 'Residualisation and council housing: aspects of the changing social relations of housing tenure', *Journal of Social Policy*, 12, 4, pp. 453–68.

—— (1994) 'Home ownership in recession', *Housing Studies*, 9, 1, pp. 55–74.

Forrest, R., Murie, A. and Williams, P. (1990) *Home Ownership: Differentiation and Fragmentation*, London: Unwin Hyman.

Foyer Federation for Youth (1998a) *Newsletter No. 3: Summer 1998*, London: FFY.

—— (1998b) *Values and Viabilities: Measuring Occupancy Levels in Foyers*, London: FFY.

Furlong, A. (1992) *Growing up in a Classless Society? School to Work Transitions*, Edinburgh: Edinburgh University Press.

Furlong, A. and Cartmel, F. (1997) *Young People and Social Change: Individualisation and Risk in Late Modernity*, Buckingham: Open University Press.

—— (forthcoming) *Youth Unemployment in Rural Areas*, York: Joseph Rowntree Foundation.

Furlong, A. and Cooney, G. (1990) 'Getting on their bikes: teenagers leaving home in Scotland in the 1980s', *Journal of Social Policy*, 19, 4, pp. 535–51.

Garnett, L. (1992) *Leaving Care and After*, London: National Children's Bureau.

Garside, P. (1993) 'Housing needs, family values and single homeless people', *Policy and Politics*, 21, 4, pp. 319–28.

Giddens, A. (1991) *Modernity and Self Identity: Self and Society in the Late Modern Age*, Cambridge: Polity Press.

Gilchrist, R. and Jeffs, T. (1995) 'Foyers: housing solution or folly?', *Youth and Policy*, 50, Autumn, pp. 1-12.

Gill, B., Meltzer, H., Hinds, K. and Petticrew, M. (1996) *Psychiatric Morbidity among Homeless People*, London: Office of National Statistics.

Goodlad, R. (1993) *The Housing Authority as Enabler*, London: Longman/Institute of Housing.

—— (1994) 'Conceptualising enabling: the housing role of local authorities', *Local Government Studies*, 20, 4, pp. 570–87.

Green, A. E. (1997) 'Employment constraints and opportunities in rural areas', *Institute for Employment Research Bulletin*, 35.

Green, A. E., Elias, P., Hogarth, T., Holmans, A., McKnight, A. and Owen, D. (1997) *Housing, Family and Working Lives*, Warwick: Institute for Employment Research.

Green, H. and Hansbro, J. (1995) *Housing in England 1993/4: A Report of the 1993/4 Survey of English Housing*, London: HMSO.

Green, H. and Holroyd, S. (1992) *Shared Accommodation in England and Wales*, London: HMSO.

Green, H., Deacon, K. and Down, D. (1998) *Housing in England 1996/7: A Report of the 1996/7 Survey of English Housing*, London: HMSO.

Green, H., Deacon, K., Iles, N. and Down, D. (1997) *Housing in England 1995/6: A Report of the 1995/6 Survey of English Housing*, London: HMSO.

Green, H., Thomas, M., Iles, N. and Down, D. (1996) *Housing in England 1994/5: A Report of the 1994/5 Survey of English Housing*, London: HMSO.

Greve, J. (1971) *Homeless in London*, London and Edinburgh: Scottish Academic Press.

Greve, J. with Currie, E. (1991) *Homelessness in Britain*, York: Joseph Rowntree Foundation.

Griffin, C. (1985) *Typical Girls: Young Women from School to the Job Market*, London: Routledge and Kegan Paul.

Griffiths, S. (1997) *Benefit Shortfalls: The Impact of Housing Benefit Cuts on Young Single People*, London: Shelter.

Hall, J. (1996) *Status Zero: a Young Person's Road to Homelessness*, London: The De Paul Trust.

Hancock, L. (1997) 'Housing chaos for new students', *Independent on Sunday*, 5 Oct.

Harding, J. and Keenan, P. (1998) 'The provision of furnished accommodation by local authorities', *Housing Studies*, 13, 3, pp. 377–90.

Hardy, F. (1994) 'A secure home? CAB evidence on housing and homelessness in London', *Occasional Paper 6*, London: NACAB.

Hardy, M. and Crow, G. (eds) (1991) *Lone Parenthood: Coping with Constraints and Making Opportunities*, Hemel Hempstead: Harvester Wheatsheaf.

Harris, S. (1989) *Social Security for Young People*, Aldershot: Avebury.

Hills, J. (1998) *Income and Wealth: the Latest Evidence*, York: Joseph Rowntree Foundation.

Holmans, A. (1995a) *Estimating the First-time Buyer Population in the United Kingdom: an Age Analysis*, London: Council of Mortgage Lenders.

—— (1995b) *Housing Need and Demand in England 1991–2011*, York: Joseph Rowntree Foundation.

Holmans, A. (1996) 'Leaving home and household formation by young men and women', in Green, H., Thomas, M., Nicola, I. and Down, D. (eds) *Housing in England 1994/5*, London: HMSO.

Holmes, C. (1998) 'Is it asking to much?', *Roof*, March/April, pp. 10–11.

Holmström, J. (1997) 'Increased homelessness in Brighton and Hove', unpublished report by the Brighton Housing Trust.

Huby, M. and Dix, G. (1992) *Evaluating the Social Fund*: London HMSO.

Hutson, S. and Jenkins, R. (1989) *Taking the Strain: Families, Unemployment and the Transition to Adulthood*, Milton Keynes: Open University Press.

Hutson, S. and Liddiard, M. (1994) *Youth Homelessness: The Construction of a Social Issue*, London: Macmillan.

Irvine, M. (1996) *The Housing Act 1996: a Guide*, Coventry: Chartered Institute of Housing (with ADC and AMA).

Jones, G. (1987) 'Leaving the parental home: an analysis of early housing careers', *Journal of Social Policy*, 16, 1, pp. 49–74.

—— (1990) *Housing Formation amongst Young Adults in Scotland*, Scottish Homes Discussion Paper 2.

—— (1991) 'The cost of living in the parental home', *Youth and Policy*, 32, pp. 19–29.

—— (1992) 'Leaving home in rural Scotland', *Youth and Policy*, 39, pp. 34–44.

—— (1995a) *Family Support for Young People*, London: Family Policy Studies Centre.

—— (1995b) *Leaving Home*, Buckingham: Open University Press.

Jones, G. and Jamieson, L. (1996) 'Young people in rural Scotland: getting out and staying on', *CES Briefing*.

Jones G. and Wallace, C. (1992) *Youth, Family and Citizenship*, Buckingham: Open University Press.

Jordan, B. (1996) *A Theory of Poverty and Social Exclusion*, Cambridge: Polity Press.

Kahn, V. and Henderson J. W. (1987) *Race, Class and state Housing: Inequality and the Allocation of Public Housing in Britain*, London: Gower.

Kay, H. (1994) *Conflicting Priorities*, London: CHAR.

Kemeny, J. (1981) *The Myth of Home Ownership*, London: Routledge and Kegan Paul.

Kemp, P. A. (1988) 'Private renting: an overview', in Kemp, P. A. (ed.) *The Private Provision of Rented Housing*, Aldershot: Avebury.

—— (1992) *Housing Benefit: an Appraisal*, London: HMSO.

—— (1997) 'Ideology, public policy and private rental housing since the war', in Williams, P. (ed.) *Directions in Housing Policy*, London: Paul Chapman Publishing.

Kemp, P. A. and Rhodes, D. (1994a) *The Lower End of the Private Rented Sector: A Glasgow Case Study*, Edinburgh: Scottish Homes.

—— (1994b) *Private Landlords in Scotland*, Edinburgh: Scottish Homes.

Kemp, P. A. and Rugg, J. (1998) *The Single Room Rent: Its Impact on Young People*, York: Centre for Housing Policy, University of York.

Kemp, P. A. and Willington, S. (1995) 'Students and the private rented sector in Scotland', *Housing Research Review*, 7, Edinburgh: Scottish Homes.

Kemp, P., Oldman, C., Rugg, J., and Williams, T. (1994) *The Effects of Benefit on Housing Decisions*, London: HMSO.

Kempson, E. and Ford, J. (1995) *Attitudes, Beliefs and Confidence: Consumer Views of the Housing Market in the 1990s*, London: Council of Mortgage Lenders.

Kiernan, K. and Wicks, M. (1990) *Family Change and Future Policy*, York: Joseph Rowntree Foundation/Family Policy Studies Centre.

Kilburn, A. (1996) 'The challenge of rural housing', *Housing Review*, 45, 2, March/April.

Killeen, D. (1992) 'Leaving home', in Coleman, J. C. and Warren-Anderson, C. (eds) *Youth Policy in the 1990s: the Way Forward*, London: Routledge.

Kirby, P. (1994) *A Word From The Street*, London: Centrepoint Soho/Community Care.

Kirk, D., Nelson, S., Sinfield, A. and Sinfield, D. (1991) *Excluding Youth: Poverty Among Young People Living Away From Home*, Edinburgh: Bridges Project/University of Edinburgh.

Kirk, N. (1997) *DSS Not Welcome: How the Housing Benefit Safety Net was Lost*, London: National Homeless Alliance.

Lash, S. and Urry, J. (1987) *The End of Organised Capitalism*, Cambridge: Polity Press.

Laslett, R. (1998) 'Will student debt damage the mortgage market?', *Housing Finance*, 37, pp. 31–6.

Lee, P. and Murie, A. (1997) *Poverty, Housing Tenure and Social Exclusion*, Bristol: The Policy Press.

Lee, P., Murie, A., Marsh, A. and Riseborough, M. (1995) *The Price of Social Exclusion*, London: National Federation of Housing Associations.

Lidstone, P. (1994) 'Rationing housing to the homeless applicant', *Housing Studies*, 9, 4, pp. 459–72.

London Research Centre (1996) *Estimates of Young Single Homelessness – A Report to NCH Action for Children*, London: NCH Action for Children.

Lowe, K. (1990) *Teenagers in Foster Care*, London: National Foster Care Association.

MacDonald, R. (ed.) (1997) *Youth, the 'Underclass' and Social Exclusion*, London: Routledge.

McCluskey, J. (1993) *Breaking the Spiral: Ten Myths on the Children Act and Youth Homelessness*, London: CHAR.

—— (1994) *Acting in Isolation: an Evaluation of the Effectiveness of the Children Act for Young Homeless People*, London: CHAR.

McDowell, L. (1978) 'Competition in the private rented sector: students and low-income families in Brighton, Sussex', *Transactions of the Institute of British Geographers*, 3, 1, pp. 55–66.

McLaughlin, B. (1986) 'The rhetoric and reality of rural deprivation', *Journal of Rural Studies*, 2, 4, pp. 291–307.

McManus, J. (1998) 'Care leavers need more help', *Working Brief*, London: Youthaid Unemployment Unit.

Maclagan, I. (1993) *Four Years' Severe Hardship: Young People and the Benefits Gap*, London: COPYSS.

Maclennan, D., Meen, G., Gibb, K. and Stephens, M. (1997) *Fixed Commitments, Uncertain Incomes: Sustainable Owner-Occupation and the Economy*, York: Joseph Rowntree Foundation.

Madge, J. and Brown, C. (1991) *First Homes: A Study of the Housing Circumstances of Young Married Couples*, London: Policy Studies Institute.

Malpass, P. and Murie. A. (1994) *Housing Policy and Practice* (4th edition), London: Macmillan.

Markey, K. (1998) 'Somewhere to call home', *The Big Issue in the North*, No. 201, March 16–22.

Marsh, A. and McKay, S. (1993) *Families, Work and Benefits*, London: Policy Studies Institute.

Marsh, A. and Riseborough, M. (1998) 'Expanding private renting: flexibility at a price?', in Marsh, A. and Mullins, D. (eds) *Housing and Public Policy: Citizenship, Choice and Control*, Buckingham: Open University Press.

Matthews, R. (1985) 'Out of house and home? The board and lodgings regulations', *Poverty*, 62, Winter.

Millham, S., Bullock, R., Hosie, K. and Haak, M. (1986) *Lost in Care*, Aldershot: Gower.

Mitchell, W. A. (1998) 'Leaving school: transition experiences and routes taken by disabled young people', unpublished D.Phil. thesis, Department of Social Policy and Social Work, University of York.

Morgan, D. and McDowell, L. (1979) *Patterns of Residence: Cost and Options in Student Housing*, Guildford: Society for Research into Higher Education.

Morrow, G. and Richards, M. (1996) *Transitions to Adulthood: a Family Matter?*, York: Joseph Rowntree Foundation.

Morton, E. (1998) *South Yorkshire: Tackling Youth Homelessness*, London: Shelter.

Mullins, D. and Niner, P. with Marsh, A. and Walker, B. (1996) *Evaluation of the 1991 Homelessness Code of Guidance*, London: HMSO.

Mullins, D., Niner, P. and Riseborough, M. (1992) *Evaluating Large Scale Voluntary Transfers of Local Authority Housing: Interim Report*, London: HMSO.

—— (1995) *Evaluating Large Scale Voluntary Transfers of Local Authority Housing*, London: HMSO.

Murie, A. (1997) 'The housing divide', in *British Social Attitudes Survey, Report No. 14*, Aldershot: Ashgate Publishing.

NACAB (1990) *Hard Times for Social Fund Applicants*, London: National Association of Citizens Advice Bureaux.

Nassor, I. (1996) *Youth Affairs Briefing*, London: Centrepoint Soho.

National Assistance Board (NAB) (1966) *Single Homeless Persons*, London: HMSO.

National Children's Bureau (1992) *Child Facts*, 25 June, London: National Children's Bureau.

National Committee of Inquiry into Higher Education (1997) *Report of the National Committee*, London: HMSO.

National Union of Students (NUS) (1996) *Accommodation Costs Survey Report 1996/97*, London: NUS.

NCH (1993) *A Lost Generation?*, London: NCH Action for Children.

Neale, J. (1997) 'Homelessness and theory reconsidered' *Housing Studies*, 4, 1, pp. 47–61.

Nicholson, L. and Wasoff, F. (1989) *Students' Experience of Private Rented Housing in Edinburgh*, Edinburgh: University of Edinburgh.

O'Callaghan, B. and Dominian, L., with Evans, A., Dix, J., Smith, R., Williams, P. and Zimmeck, M. (1996) *Study of Homeless Applicants*, London: HMSO.

OECD (1996) *Beyond 2000: The New Social Policy Agenda*, Conference issues paper.

Office of National Statistics (1998) Information on the population of the UK provided on the ONS website, http://www.ons.gov.uk/

Oxley, A. (1993) *Not me! Housing Education: The Case for Preventive Medicine*, Leeds: Yorkshire Metropolitan Housing Association.

Packman, J. and Jordan, B. (1991) 'The Children Act: looking forward, looking back', *Children and Society*, 21, 4, pp. 315–27.

Parker, J., Smith, R. and Williams, P. (1992) *Access, Allocations and Nominations: the Role of Housing Associations*, London: HMSO.

Parton, N. (1991) *Governing the Family: Child Care, Child Protection and the state*, Basingstoke: Macmillan.

Pawson, H. and Third, H. (1997) 'Spot the difference', *Inside Housing*, 12 September.

Pierce, N. and Hillman, J. (1998) *Wasted Youth: Raising Achievement and Tackling Social Exclusion*, London: IPPR.

Pleace, N. (1995) *Housing Single Vulnerable Homeless People*, York: Centre for Housing Policy, University of York.

—— (1998a) *The Open House Programme for People Sleeping Rough: An Evaluation*, York: Centre for Housing Policy.

—— (1998b) 'Single homelessness as social exclusion: the unique and the extreme' *Social Policy and Administration*, 32, 1, pp. 46–59.

Pleace, N. and Quilgars, D. (1996) *Health and Homelessness in London: A Review*, London: The King's Fund.

Pleace, N., Ford, J., Wilcox, S. and Burrows, R. (1998) *Lettings and Sales by Registered Social Landlords 1996/97*, London: Housing Corporation.

Ploeg, J. van der and Scholte, E. (1997) *Homeless Youth*, London: Sage.

Power, A. and Tunstall, R. (1995) *Swimming Against the Tide: Polarisation or Progress on 30 Unpopular Estates, 1980–95*, York: Joseph Rowntree Foundation.

—— (1997) *Dangerous Disorder: Riots and Violent Disturbances in Thirteen Areas of Britain, 1991-2*, York: Joseph Rowntree Foundation.

Prescott-Clarke, P., Allen, P. and Morrissey, C. (1988) *Queuing for Housing: a Study of Council Housing Waiting Lists*, London: HMSO.

Prescott-Clarke, P., Clemens, S. and Park, A. (1994) *Routes into Local Authority Housing: A Study of Local Authority Waiting Lists and New Tenancies*, London: HMSO.

Prime, D. (1998) *Crawley and Horsham: Tackling Youth Homelessness*, London: Shelter.

Quilgars, D. and Anderson, I. (1997) 'Addressing the problem of youth homelessness and unemployment: the contribution of foyers', in Burrows, R., Pleace, N. and Quilgars, D. (eds) *Homelessness and Social Policy*, London: Routledge.

Randall, G. (1988) *No Way Home*, London: Centrepoint Soho.

—— (1989) *Homeless and Hungry*, London: Centrepoint.

Randall, G. and Brown, S. (1993) *The Rough Sleepers Initiative: an Evaluation*, London: HMSO.

—— (1995) *Outreach and Resettlement Work with People Sleeping Rough*, London: Department of the Environment.

—— (1996) *From Street to Home: an Evaluation of Phase 2 of the Rough Sleepers Initiative*, London: HMSO.

Residential Renting (1997) 'Housing Benefit', February.

Resource Information Service (RIS) (1998) *London Hostels Directory 1998*, London: Resource Information Service.

Rhodes, D. and Bevan, M. (1997) *Can the Private Rented Sector House the Homeless?*, York: Centre for Housing Policy, University of York.

Rhodes, D. and Kemp, P. A. (1998) *Joseph Rowntree Foundation Index of Private Rents and Yields: Fourth Quarter 1997*, York: Centre for Housing Policy, University of York.

Roberts, K. (1993) 'Career trajectories and the mirage of social mobility', in Bates, I. and Risborough, G. (eds) *Youth and Inequality*, Buckingham: Oxford University Press.

—— (1995) *Youth and Employment in Modern Britain*, London: Longman.

Robinson, G. (1992) 'The provision of rural housing: policies in the United Kingdom', in Bowler, I. R., Bryant, C. R. and Nellis, N. D. (eds) *Contemporary Rural Systems in Transition: Vol. 2 Economy and Society*, Oxford: CAB International.

Robson, P. and Poustie, M. (1996) *Homeless People and the Law*, London: Butterworth.

Roll, J. (1990) *Young People: Growing up in the Welfare state*, London: Family Policy Studies Centre.

Room, G. (ed.) (1995) *Beyond the Threshold. The Measurement and Analysis of Social Exclusion*, Bristol: Policy Press.

Rooney, B. (1997) *An Evaluation of Furnished Housing in Mainstream Practice*, Bristol: Policy Press and Joseph Rowntree Foundation.

Rosenbaum, M. and Bailey, J. (1991) 'Movement within England and Wales during the 1980s, as measured by the NHS central register', *Population Trends*, 65, 3, pp. 24–34.

Rosser, M. (1997) 'Home ownership and graduates', *Housing Finance*, 37, pp. 31–3.

Rugg, J. (1996) *Opening Doors: Helping People on Low Income Secure Private Rented Accommodation*, York: Centre for Housing Policy, University of York.

—— (1997) *Closing Doors? Access Schemes and the Recent Housing Changes*, York: Centre for Housing Policy, University of York.

Rugg, J., Willington, S. and Rhodes, D. (1995) 'Students and the private rented sector in York', unpublished report to the Bursar's Office, University of York.

Rural Development Commission (RDC) (1993) 'The rural housing problem', *RDC Policy Information*, November.

—— (1994a) *Rural Services: Challenges and Opportunities*, Salisbury: Rural Development Commission.

—— (1994b) *Rural Development Strategy for the 1990s*, Salisbury: Rural Development Commission.

Ruxton, S. and Burgess, A. (1996) *Men and Their Children: Proposals for Public Policy*, London: Institute of Public Policy Research.

Saunders, P. (1990) *A Nation of Home Owners*, London: Unwin Hyman.

Scottish Office Development Department (1997a) *Code of Guidance on Homelessness*, Edinburgh: Scottish Office Development Department.

—— (1997b) 'New statutory homelessness priority need group', Circular to all holders of Code of Guidance on Homelessness, 22 December.

Secretary of State for Social Services (1985a) *The Reform of Social Security: A Programme for Action*, White Paper, Command Paper 9691, London: HMSO.

—— (1985b) *Reform of Social Security – vol. 2: Programme for Change*, Command Paper 9518, London: HMSO.

Shucksmith, M., Henderson, M., Raybould, S., Coombes, M. and Wong, C. (1995) *A Classification of Rural Housing Markets in England*, London: HMSO.

Simmons, M. (1997) *Landscapes of Poverty: Aspects of Rural England in the late 1990s*, London: Lemos and Crane.

Simons, R. L. and Whitbeck, L. B. (1991) 'Running away during adolescence as a precursor to adult homelessness', *Social Services Review*, June.

Simpson, B., McCarthy, P. and Walker, J. (1995) *Being There: Fathers after Divorce*, Newcastle upon Tyne: Relate Centre for Family Studies.

Skeggs, B. (1990) 'Gender reproduction and further education: domestic apprenticeships', in Gleeson, D. (ed.) *Training and its Alternatives*, Milton Keynes: Open University Press.

—— (1997) *Formations of Class and Gender*, London: Sage.

Smith, J., Gilford, S. and O'Sullivan, A. (1998) *The Family Background of Homeless Young People*, London: Family Policy Studies Centre/Joseph Rowntree Foundation.

Smith, J., Gilford, S., Kirby, P., O'Reilly, A. and Ing, P. (1996) *Bright Lights and Homelessness*, London: YMCA.

Social Exclusion Unit (1998) *Rough Sleeping: Report by the Social Exclusion Unit*, Cmmd. 4008, London: HMSO.

Social Security Advisory Committee (1997) *The Housing Benefit and Council Tax Benefit (General) Amendment Regulations 1997*, Command Paper 3598, London: HMSO.

Social Services Inspectorate (1997) *When Leaving Home is also Leaving Care: An Inspection of Services for Young People Leaving Care*, Wetherby: Department of Health.

Sone, K. (1994) 'Home of their own', *Community Care*, 6–12 October.

Spafford, J. (1994) *Centrepoint Oxfordshire: a Regional Approach to a National Problem*, London: Centrepoint.

Speak, S. (1998) *The Employment Situation of Young Single Parent from Disadvantaged Neighbourhoods*, Newcastle upon Tyne: Department of Town and Country Planning, University of Newcastle upon Tyne.

Speak, S., Gilroy, R. and Cameron, S. (1997) *Young Single Fathers: their Participation in Fatherhood*, London: Family Policy Studies Centre.

Speak, S., Gilroy, R., Cameron, S. and Woods, R. (1995) *Young Single Mothers: Barriers to Independent Living*, London: Family Policy Studies Centre.

Spittles, D. (1997) 'Welcome to the Hotel Academia', *Evening Standard*, 7 May.

Steel, J. and Sausman, C. (1997) *The Contribution of Graduates to the Economy: Rates of Return*, Report No. 7, The National Committee of Enquiry into Higher Education, London: HMSO.

Stein, M. (1991) *Leaving Care and the 1989 Children Act: The Agenda*, Leeds: First Key.

Stein, M. and Carey, K. (1986) *Leaving Care*, Oxford: Blackwell.

Stern, E. and Turbin, J. (1986) *Youth Employment and Unemployment in Rural England*, Salisbury: Rural Development Commission.

Stone, I. (1998) *Lincolnshire: Tackling Youth Homelessness*, London: Shelter.

Strathdee, R. (1992) *No Way Back*, London: Centrepoint Soho.

—— (1993) *Housing Our Children: the Children Act 1989*, London: Centrepoint Soho.

Strathdee, R. and Johnson, M. (1994) *Out of Care and on the Streets: Young People, Care Leavers and Homelessness*, London: Centrepoint.

Taylor, M. with Wainwright, S. (1996) 'Stock transfer', in Currie. H. and Murie, A. (eds) *Housing in Scotland*, Coventry: Chartered Institute of Housing.

Thane, P. (1989) *The Foundations of the Welfare State*, London: Longman.

Thomas, A., Snape, D., Duldig, W., Keegan, J. and Ward, K. (1995) *In from the Cold – Working with the Private Landlord*, London: Department of the Environment.

Trickett, L. (1995) *Landlord and Agent Survey: Implications for the Private Rented Sector*, Birmingham: Birmingham City Council.

Turbin, J. and Stern, E. (1987) 'Rural youth labour markets', in Brown, P. and Ashton, D. N. (eds) *Education, Unemployment and Labour Markets*, Lewes: Falmer Press.

Venn, S. (1985) *Singled Out: Local Authority Housing Policies for Single People*, London: CHAR.

Vincent, J., Deacon, A. and Walker, R. (1995) *Homeless Single Men: Roads to Resettlement?*, Aldershot: Avebury.

Wade, J. and Biehal, N. with Clayden, J. and Stein, M. (1998) *Going Missing: Young People Absent from Care*, Chichester, Wiley.

Wallace, C. (1987) *For Richer, for Poorer: Growing Up In and Out of Work*, London: Tavistock.

Watson, S. and Austerberry, H. (1986) *Housing and Homelessness: a Feminist Perspective*, London: Routledge and Kegan Paul.

Whitehead, C. and Kleinman, M. (1992) *A Review of Housing Needs Assessment*, London: Housing Corporation.

Wilcox, S. (1996) *Housing Review 1996/7*, York: Joseph Rowntree Foundation.

—— (1997) *Housing Finance Review 1997/8*, York: Joseph Rowntree Foundation.

Williams, P. (ed.) (1997) *Directions in Housing Policy*, London: Paul Chapman.

Williamson, H. (1997) 'Status zero, youth and the "underclass": some considerations' in MacDonald, R. (ed.) *Youth, the Underclass and Social Exclusion*, London: Routledge.

Withers, P. and Randolph, B. (1994) *Access, Homelessness and Housing Associations*, Research Report 21, London: NFHA.

Young Homelessness Group (1991) *Carefree and Homeless*, London: Young Homelessness Group.

Zijl, V. van (1993) *A Guide to Local Housing Needs Assessment*, Coventry: Institute of Housing.

Index